Yoga Se Hi Hoga

101 Benefits of Yoga

©VARUNA SACHETI

NOTION PRESS

NOTION PRESS

India. Singapore. Malaysia.

This book has been published with all reasonable efforts taken to make the material error-free after the consent of the author. No part of this book shall be used, reproduced in any manner whatsoever without written permission from the author, except in the case of brief quotations embodied in critical articles and reviews.

The Author of this book is solely responsible and liable for its content including but not limited to the views, representations, descriptions, statements, information, opinions and references ["Content"]. The Content of this book shall not constitute or be construed or deemed to reflect the opinion or expression of the Publisher or Editor. Neither the Publisher nor Editor endorse or approve the Content of this book or guarantee the reliability, accuracy or completeness of the Content published herein and do not make any representations or warranties of any kind, express or implied, including but not limited to the implied warranties of merchantability, fitness for a particular purpose. The Publisher and Editor shall not be liable whatsoever for any errors, omissions, whether such errors or omissions result from negligence, accident, or any other cause or claims for loss or damages of any kind, including without limitation, indirect or consequential loss or damage arising out of use, inability to use, or about the reliability, accuracy or sufficiency of the information contained in this book

To the love of my life Mr Sahil Kothari - CA
This book is a testament to the unwavering support, boundless love, and endless encouragement you have showered upon me. Through every chapter of our life together, you've been my rock, my muse, and my greatest inspiration. Your belief in me has fueled my creativity, and your presence has filled my world with joy.

I dedicate this book to my daughter To my beloved daughter, Jashvi Kothari. Your presence in my life has added depth, purpose, and a profound sense of wonder. As you hold this book in your hands, I hope it serves as a testament to the limitless potential within you. May it inspire you to chase your dreams, embrace challenges, and never stop exploring the vast world of knowledge and imagination.

This dedication is a tribute to my sister Jagrati Sacheti - Associate Manager in an Automation company; for the unwavering bond we share, the countless memories we've created, and the love that grows stronger with each passing day. Thank you for being my confidant, my partner-in-crime, and my source of endless joy. With all my love and gratitude.

This book is also dedicated to my parents and my in laws Your unwavering love, endless encouragement, and the values you instilled in me have been the guiding light on my journey as an author. This book is a testament to your endless support and belief in my dreams. Thank you for always being my biggest champions.

Contents

Foreword

Varuna Sacheti hails from the picturesque City of Lakes, Udaipur, where she spent her formative years. She earned her Bachelor's degree in Electronics & Communication Engineering from Geetanjali Institute of Technical Studies, affiliated with Rajasthan Technical University.

With a robust professional background spanning 8 years, Varuna embarked on her entrepreneurial journey in 2020 when she joined the renowned fitness community, FITTR, as a FITTR Personal Training (PT) coach.

In 2021, Varuna furthered her expertise by obtaining a Diploma in Fitness & Nutrition from the Indian Institute of Fitness and Science (INFS) Pune, in addition to completing certificate courses in Yoga from both INFS and the Yoga Certification Board (YCB), an initiative under the Ayush Ministry of the Government of India.

Over the years, Varuna has developed a strong rapport with more than 100 clients hailing from over 5 different countries. Some of these clients have been under her guidance for nearly a year, a testament to her commitment and effectiveness.

Varuna is a firm believer in the transformative, healing, rejuvenating, restorative, and uplifting qualities of yoga. She is motivated by the desire to support and inspire individuals to step onto their yoga mats and continue to do so, confident that through this practice, she is contributing positively to their lives.

Varuna's journey is a testament to the courage to follow one's dreams, even amidst challenges. With her daughter Jashvi's inspiration, Varuna's story underscores the profound effect of pursuing passions.

This book captures Varuna Sacheti's remarkable odyssey, motivating readers to embrace change and follow their own aspirations.

vi

Author: KHUSHBOO BHAVESH CHOTALIYA

Founder – Sanskari Decor (Wedding Decor Exporter) & Author

Date: September 2nd, 2023

Gratitude

I am immensely grateful to my mentor, my Digital Leadership Trainer –**Mr. Yogesh M. A**. whose timely and perceptive suggestion has ignited a transformative journey in my life - the journey of writing this book.

It was his insightful guidance that planted the seed of possibility within me, nudging me to embark on this creative endeavour.

Throughout this process, Yogesh's unwavering support has been like a guiding star, lighting up my path whenever I encountered challenges or uncertainties. His wisdom, gained from his own experiences, has been an invaluable resource, offering me both practical advice and heartfelt encouragement.

His suggestion lead to not only the creation of a book; but also personal growth and self-discovery. Writing this book became an exploration of my thoughts, insights, and passions, and I owe this enriching experience to the spark that my mentor ignited within me.

I extend my deepest appreciation to Yogesh sir. Without his pivotal suggestion and unwavering belief in me, "Yoga Se Hi Hoga" would not have come to fruition. This book stands as a testament to his profound influence and a token of my heartfelt gratitude.

Yogesh M.A. is a Digital Leadership Trainer and he has a vision of helping, guiding and encouraging 10,000+ business owners to write their own book.

He teaches Various Digital Leadership Programs for Super Busy Business Owners. You can check here www.Classroom.co.in

Thank you Yogesh M.A. sir, from the bottom of my heart.

I would also like to thank **Khushboo Chotaliya** for being my Accountability Partner for this book.

Along with her husband, Khushboo is running a company called "Sanskari Decor". They are India's leading Manufacturer, Supplier and Exporter of Wedding/Events Decor props and products. They are exporting their products to more than 10 countries.

Khushboo is on a mission of building a community of 1 Million Wedding Industry Business Owners across the globe. For that she started her International Weddings Lifestyles Talk Show named "Weddings Vista" in 2021 to support and promote Early Adaptor Business owners, Entrepreneurs and Professionals related to Wedding Industry. Khushboo hosts her talk show on a YouTube channel named "Khushboo Chotaliya". Till now Khushboo has featured 250+ business owners on her Talk Show and aims to feature 1001 business owners by 31st December 2023.

In Sept 2023, she authored her book "Weddings Vista" with the aim to impact 12.8 Million readers with the list of affirmations to bring positivity with their immediate family members.

Khushboo has contributed a lot to my Entrepreneurial journey. I am blessed to have her constant support and great encouragement.

Introduction

Welcome to a journey that holds the promise of profound transformation and well-being. In the midst of our bustling lives, where stress and uncertainty abound, the ancient art of yoga emerges as a guiding light towards a healthier, happier existence. This book, "Yoga se hi hoga", is an exploration of the incredible advantages that yoga brings to every corner of our being.

As we navigate the demands of modern existence, the wisdom of yoga becomes increasingly relevant. This book aims to serve as a comprehensive guide, shedding light on the multifaceted advantages that yoga brings to individuals of all ages and backgrounds. From enhanced flexibility and strength to inner tranquillity and mindfulness, to nurturing our minds with clarity and calm, the benefits of yoga are as diverse as they are impactful.

This book is not just a collection of facts; it's a personal journey. Drawing from my own experiences and research, I invite you to join me in uncovering the hidden gems that yoga offers. Together, we will learn how the simple act of connecting breath to movement can uplift our spirits, how the art of stillness can quiet our minds, and how the age-old wisdom of yoga can guide us towards a more harmonious life.

Whether you're a curious beginner or a seasoned practitioner, the revelations within these pages are meant to ignite your passion for yoga and its myriad benefits. So, let's begin this expedition of self-discovery, and may it lead us to a place of wellness, serenity, and a deeper connection with ourselves.

Namaste.

BENEFITS OF YOGA

Yoga, an ancient practice has become increasingly popular for today's busy and stressful world.

Yoga word is derived from the word 'YUJ' means to unite, I.e. uniting or connecting yourself 'true self' to divine essence 'atman'.

The ultimate goal of any yoga practice is to attain moksha, meaning liberation or freedom.

The eight limbs of yoga are:
• Yama - restraints
• Niyama - observations
• Asana - posture
• Pranayama - breathing practices
• Pratyahara - withdrawing the senses
• Dharana - concentration
• Dhyana - meditation
• Samadhi – enlightenment

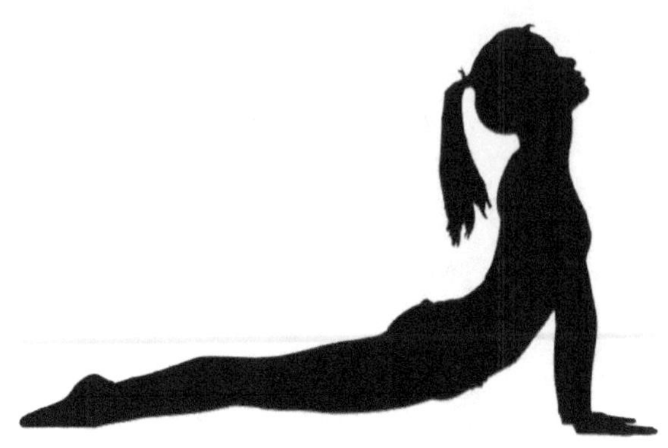

1. Yoga improves flexibility by stretching muscles and reducing tension. This leads to improved range of motion in joints, which can prevent injury and alleviate pain.

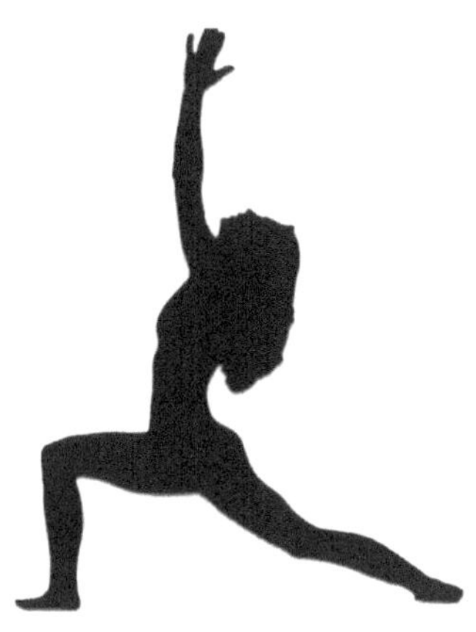

2. Yoga poses require holding positions for extended periods, which increases muscular endurance and cardiovascular health. Better endurance can improve overall physical performance.

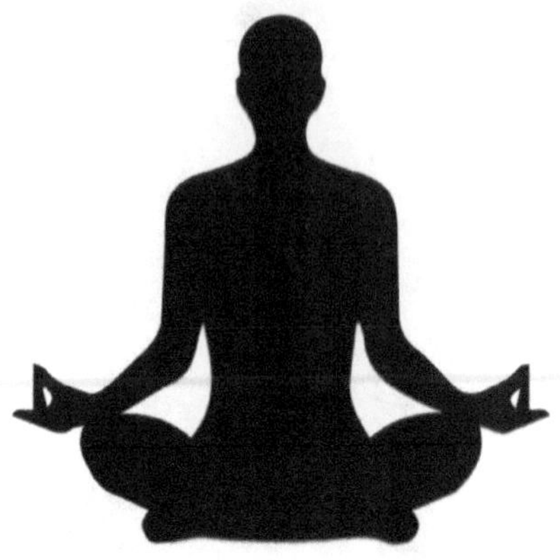

3.Yoga improves respiratory system by strengthening the respiratory muscles, improving lung capacity and promoting deep breathing.

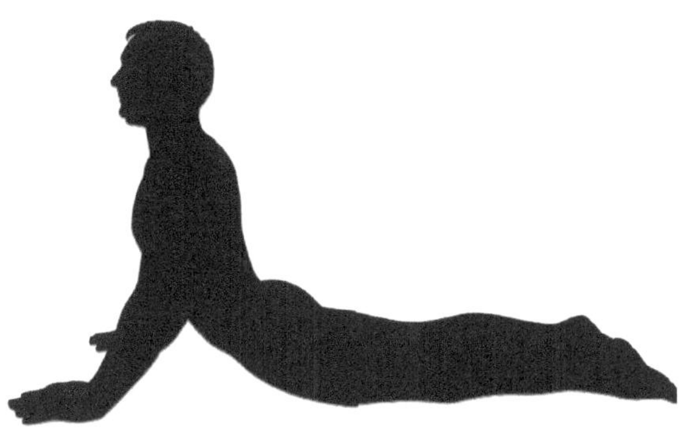

4. Yoga helps with gastrointestinal problems by stimulating digestion, reducing stress-related gut issues, and improving overall gut health through the activation of the parasympathetic nervous system.

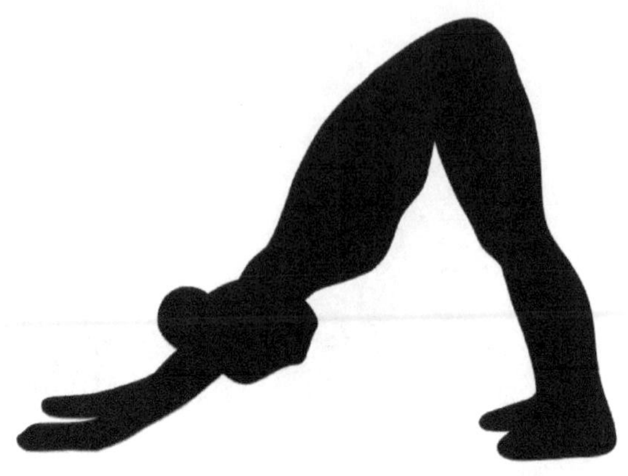

5.Yoga can help reduce menopause problems by relieving symptoms such as hot flashes, mood swings, and sleep disturbances, while also promoting relaxation, hormone balance, and overall well-being during this transitional phase.

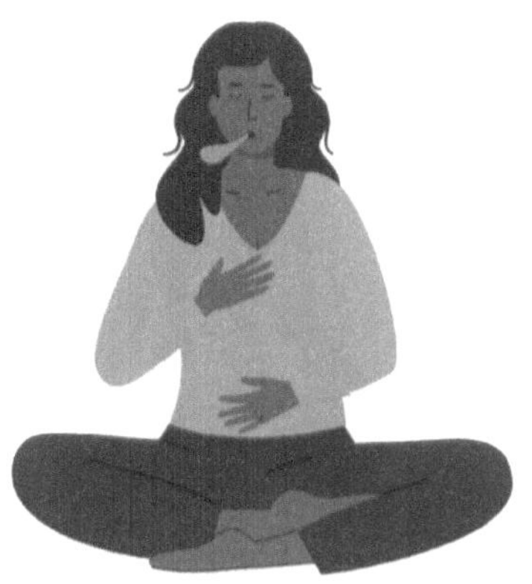

6.Pranayam & Meditation can help with patience and stress management by fostering mindfulness, promoting relaxation.

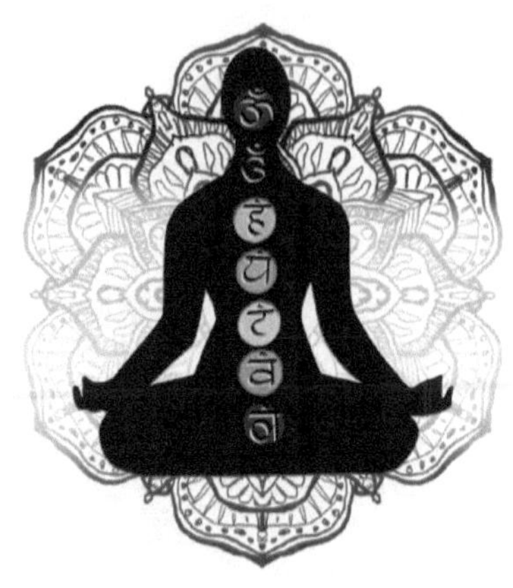

7. Yoga can increase energy levels by improving circulation, reducing stress, and promoting deep breathing, which increases oxygen flow to the body. Regular yoga practice can also stimulate the energy channels in the body, balance the chakras, and rejuvenate both the body and mind, resulting in increased vitality and energy.

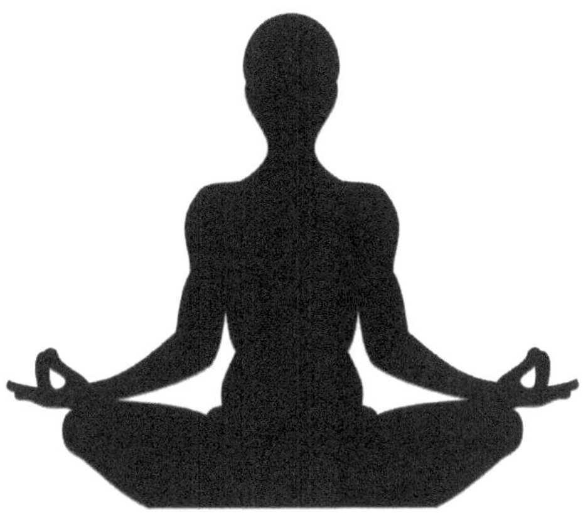

8. Pranayam & Meditation can enhance creativity and innovation by calming the mind, reducing mental clutter, and promoting a state of relaxation and receptiveness. Through breathwork, meditation, and mindful movement, yoga can help individuals tap into their creative potential, cultivate new perspectives, and unlock innovative ideas by quieting the busy mind and fostering a more open and creative mindset.

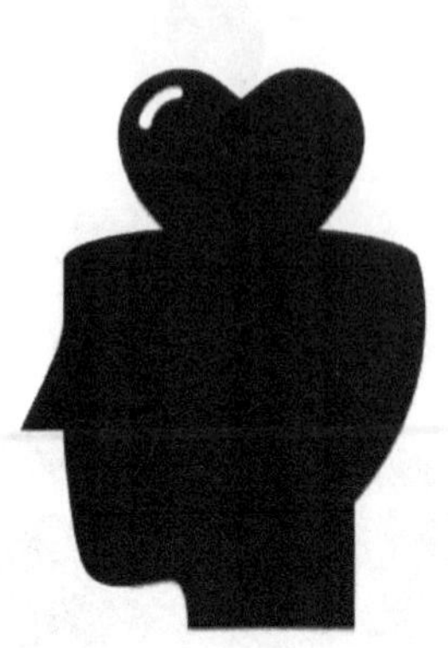

9.Yoga promotes relaxation by reducing stress and anxiety. Practicing yoga can lead to a calmer and more centered mind, which can lead to better sleep and a happier mood.

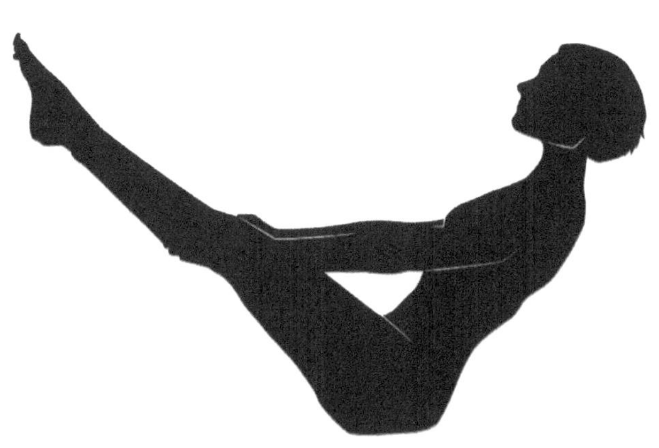

10.   Yoga can improve posture by strengthening core muscles and stretching the spine. This can help prevent back pain and reduce the risk of injury from poor posture.

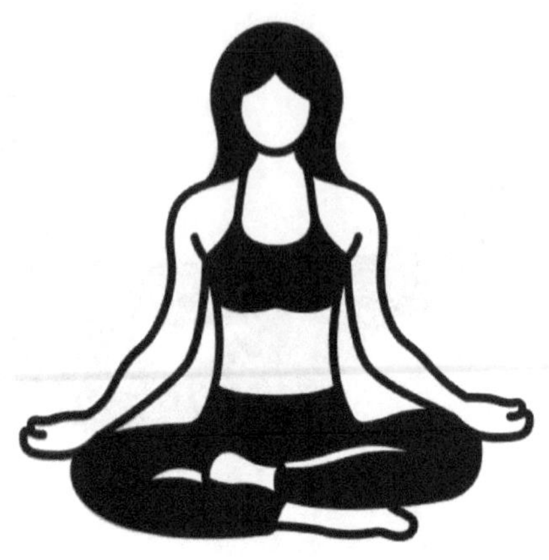

11.   Yoga has been shown to improve brain function, including cognitive performance, memory, and concentration. These benefits can lead to improved productivity and mental clarity.

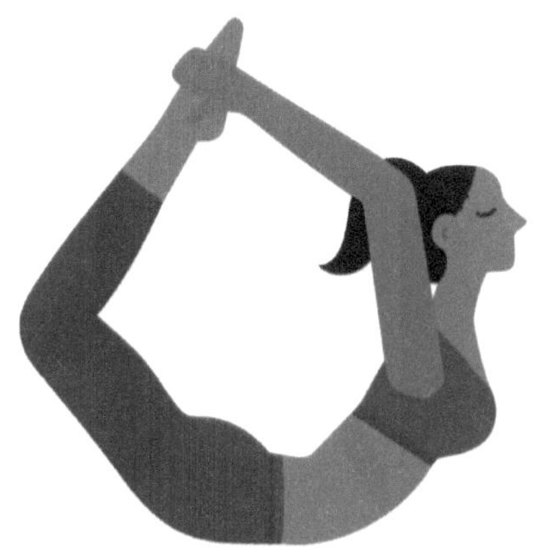

12.   Enhances self-awareness:. Practicing yoga can increase self-awareness by promoting mindfulness and introspection. This can lead to greater self-knowledge and improved decision making.

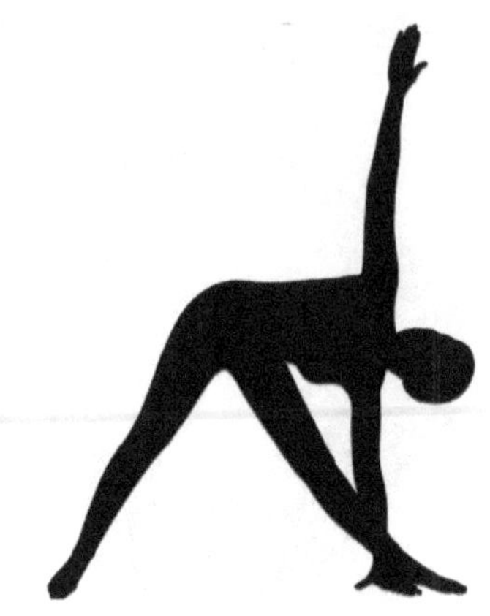

13. Yoga can improve cardiovascular health by reducing blood pressure, lowering cholesterol levels, and improving circulation. This can reduce the risk of heart disease and stroke.

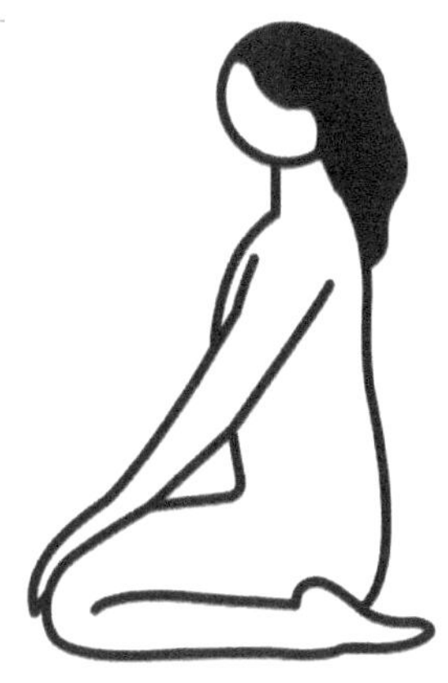

14.   Yoga has been shown to reduce inflammation in the body, which can alleviate chronic pain, improve joint health, and reduce the risk of chronic diseases such as diabetes, heart disease, and arthritis.

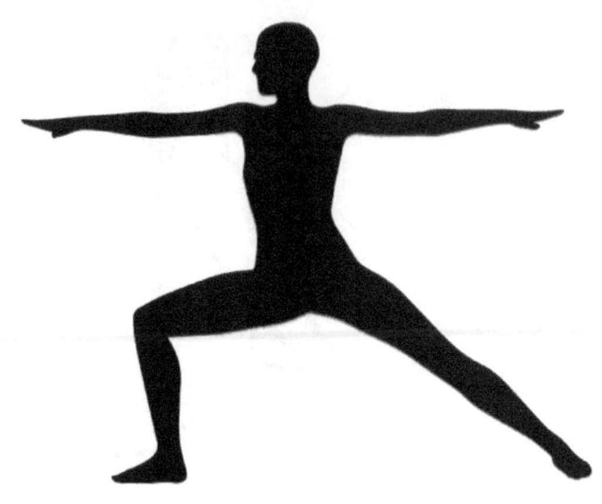

15. Yoga can promote weight loss by boosting metabolism, reducing stress, and improving digestion. It can also increase muscle mass, which burns more calories than fat.

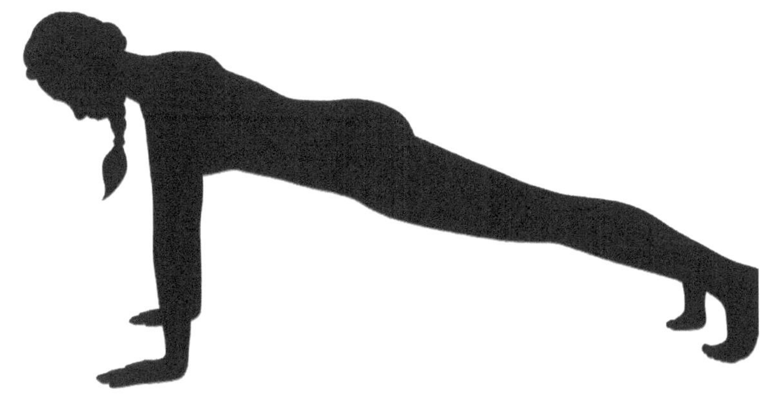

16. Yoga can alleviate joint and muscle pain by stretching and strengthening muscles, improving joint mobility, and reducing inflammation.

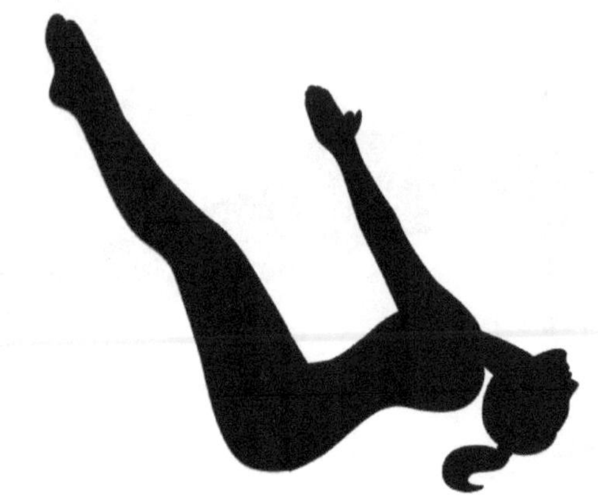

17.　Enhances immune system function: Yoga can enhance immune system function by reducing stress and boosting overall health. This can lead to better disease resistance and faster recovery from illnesses.

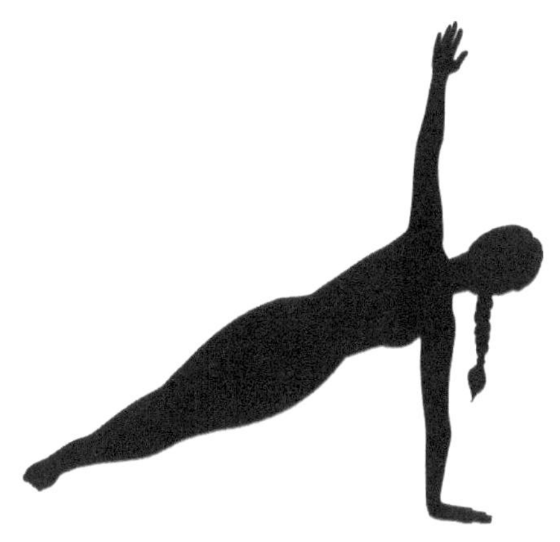

18.   Yoga asanas can improve proprioception, which is your body's awareness of its position in space. Practicing yoga postures can enhance this sense, leading to better balance and coordination in daily activities.

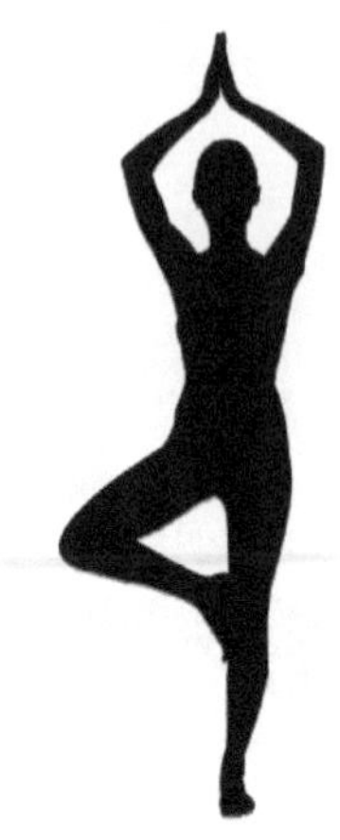

19.   Yoga poses require balance and coordination, which improve with practice. Better balance and coordination can reduce the risk of falls and improve overall physical performance.

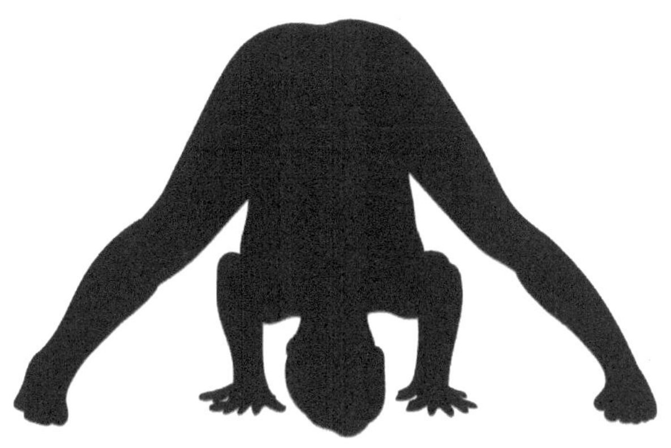

20.   Yoga poses, especially inversions like shoulder stands, can stimulate the lymphatic system, helping to detoxify the body and boost immune function.

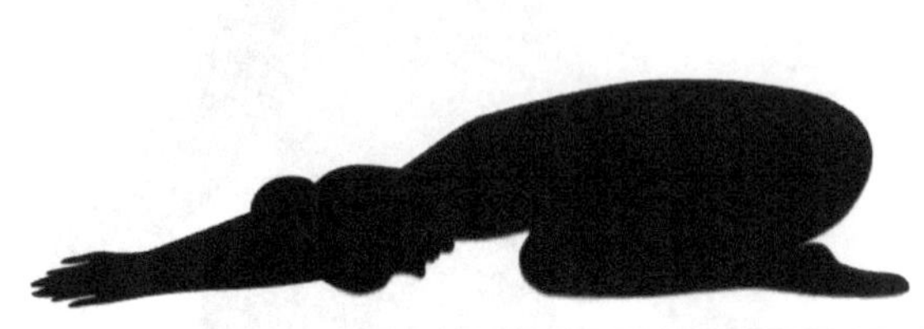

21.   Yoga can enhance creativity by relaxing the mind and allowing for fresh ideas and inspiration to flow.

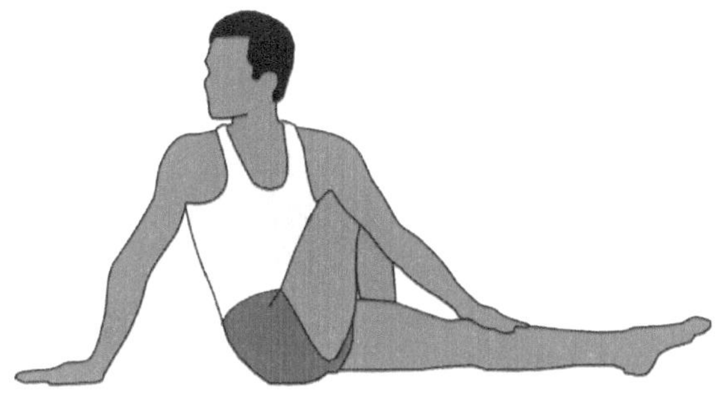

22.   Yoga can enhance lung capacity by improving respiratory function, increasing endurance, and reducing stress. This can improve overall physical performance and reduce the risk of respiratory diseases.

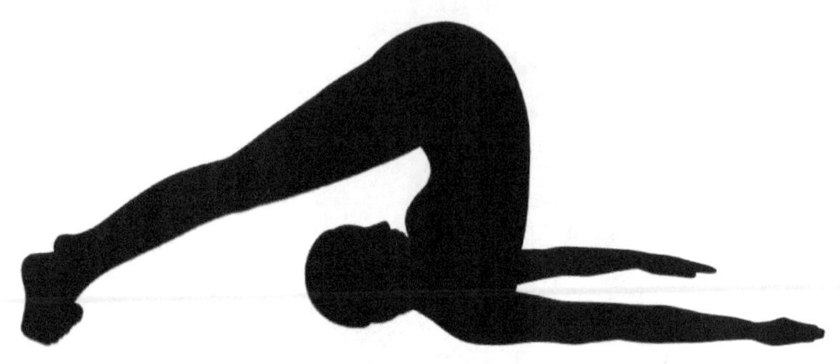

23. Yoga can reduce symptoms of depression by promoting relaxation, reducing stress, and improving brain function. It can also improve mood and overall well-being.

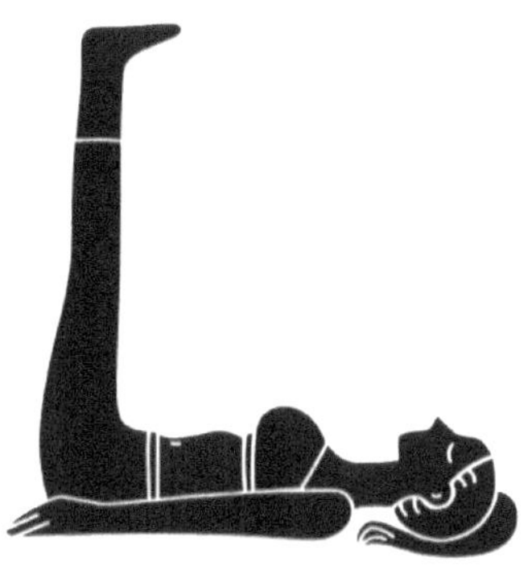

24.   Yoga postures combined with relaxation techniques can lead to more restful and deep sleep, helping to combat insomnia.

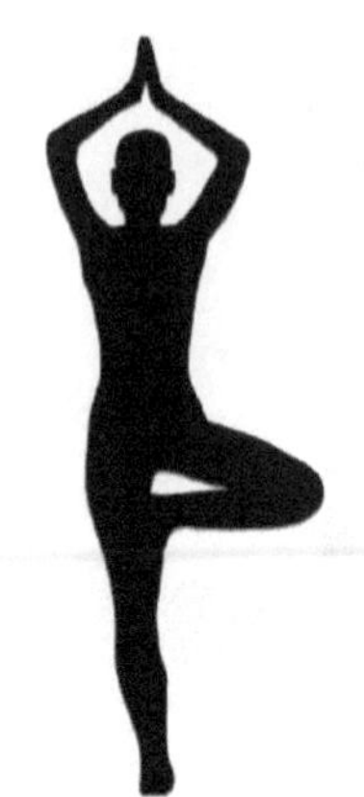

25. Yoga can promote healthy aging by reducing the risk of chronic diseases, improving mobility, and enhancing overall physical and mental health.

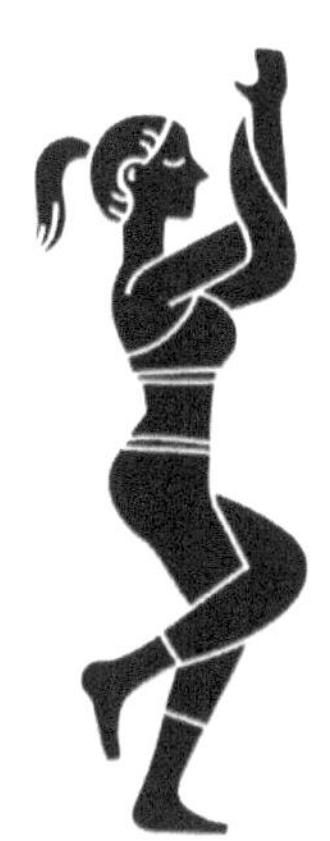

26.   Some yoga asanas and breathing exercises can help improve sexual function, increase libido and desire by increasing blood flow and reducing stress.

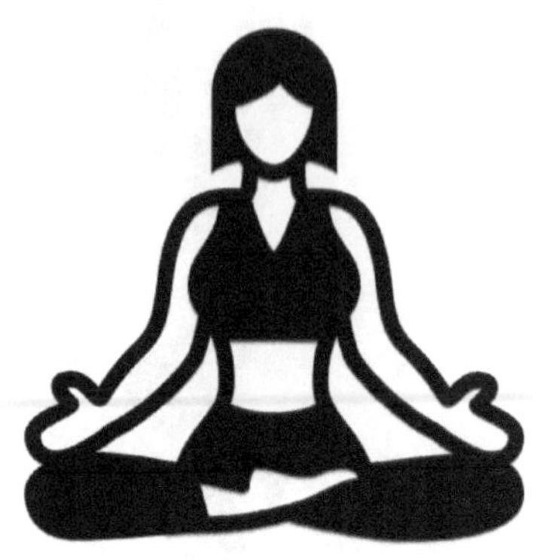

27. Yoga has a strong spiritual aspect that can enhance spiritual aspect that can enhance spiritual growth and lead to greater self-awareness and self-acceptance.

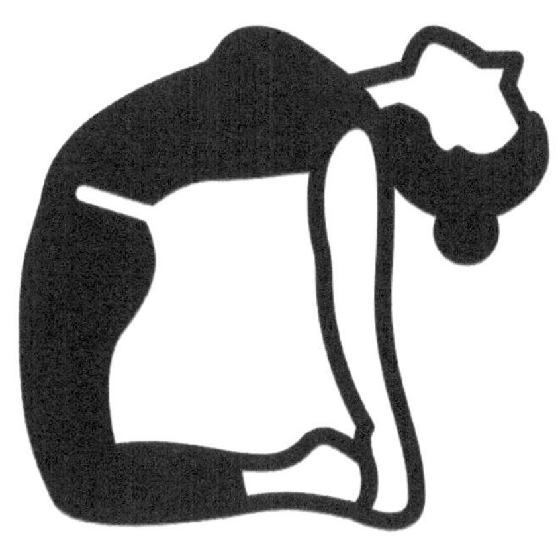

28.   In Ayurvedic medicine, yoga asanas are used to balance the doshas (body energies), promoting overall health and well-being.

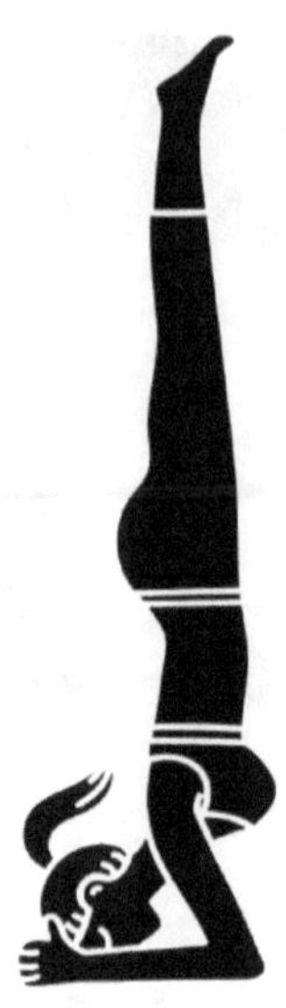

29. Yoga can enhance intuition and self-awareness by connecting the mind and body on a deeper level.

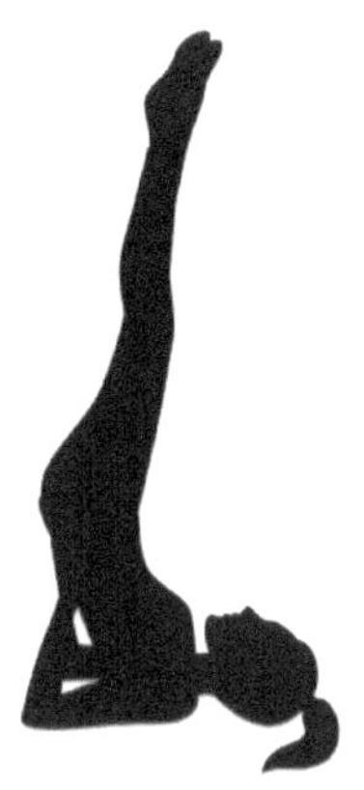

30.   Regular yoga practice, including poses that involve concentration, may improve memory and cognitive function.

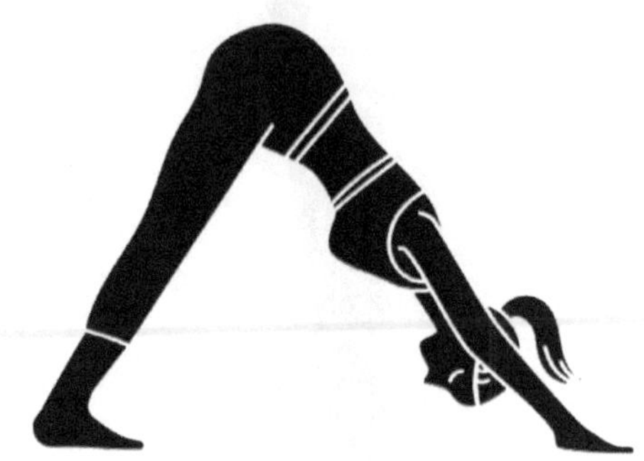

31.   Yoga improves overall posture and alignment in daily activities

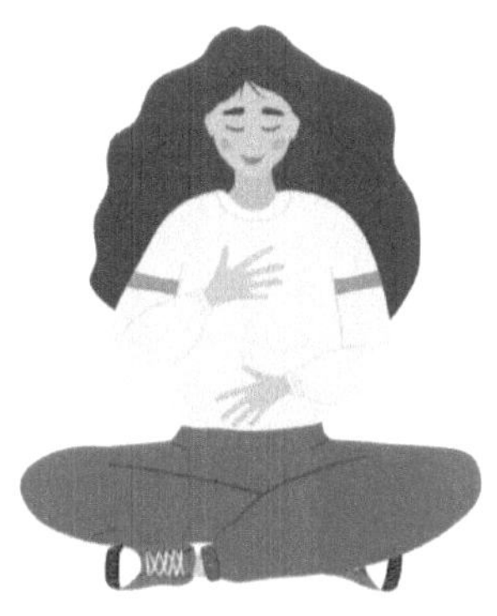

32.   YOGIC BREATHING helps in improved vitality, we are less susceptible to minor illness such as bronchitis and asthma. It Soothes & Relaxes our Nervous system.

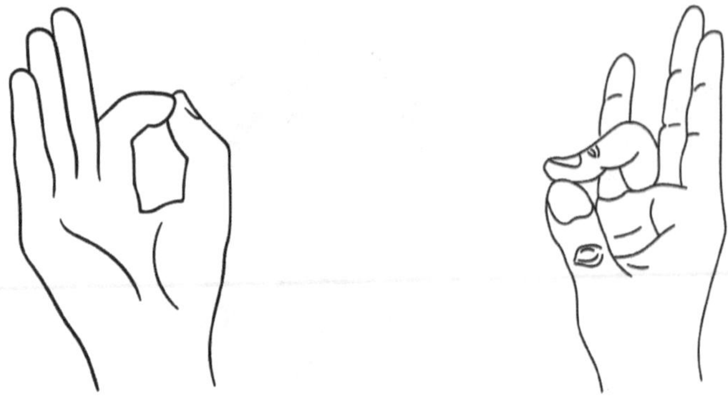

33.   To hold certain Mudras it helps improving concentration Power and memory.

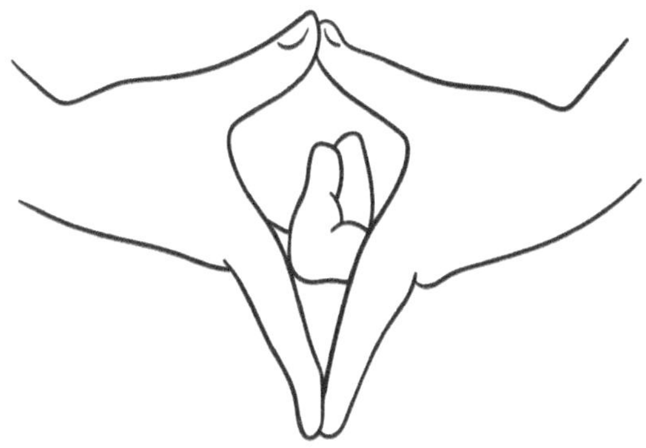

34. Yogic Mudras helps to manifest balance in fine elements- air, water, fire, earth, space and help to regain health.

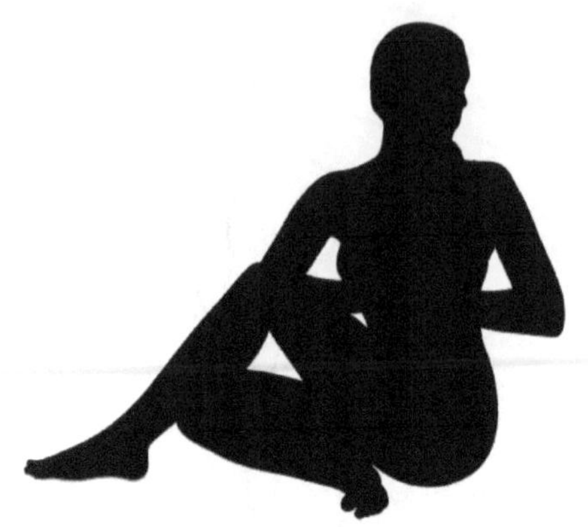

35. Regular practice of Yoga can help in decreasing blood sugar levels

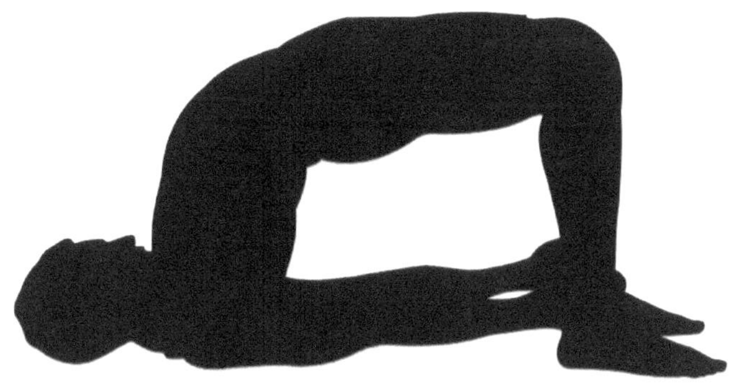

36. Yoga helps for balancing all hormonal disorders by improving Endocrine System functions.

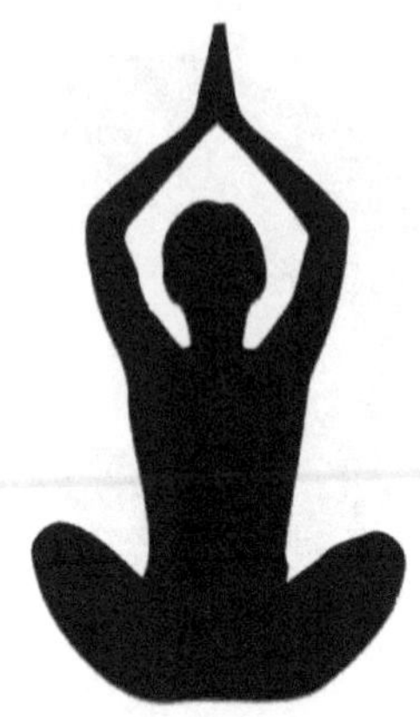

37.　Just a few minutes of yoga a day will enhance your overall wellness. You will attain a natural glow on the outside and see your body transform on the inside.

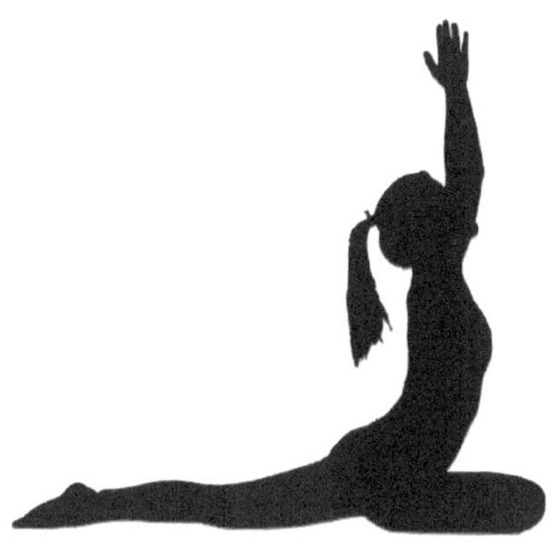

38.   Practicing yoga in group settings can foster a sense of community and improve social interactions.

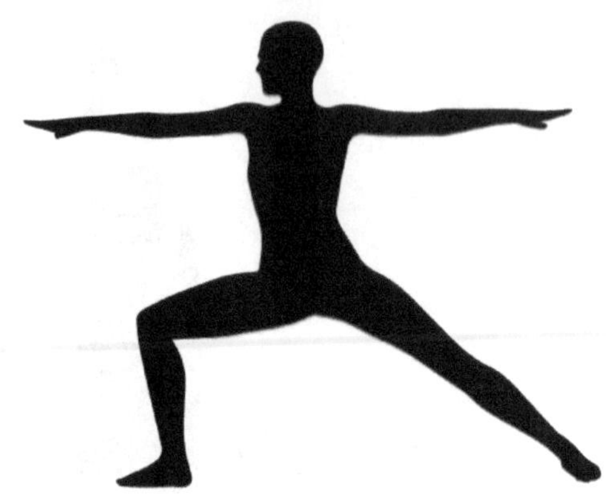

39. Yoga helps in alleviation of symptoms related to multiple sclerosis

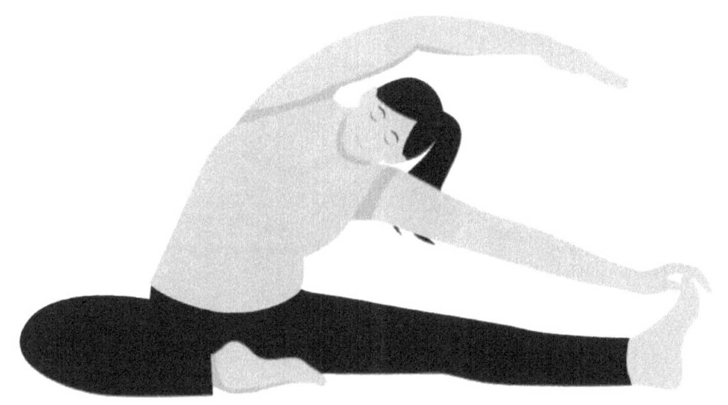

40. Yoga is known to lower blood pressure and slow the heart rate.

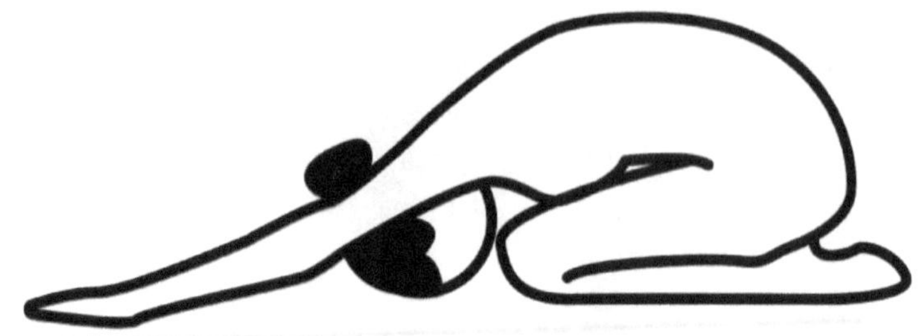

41.   It helps in better management of Chronic pain conditions.

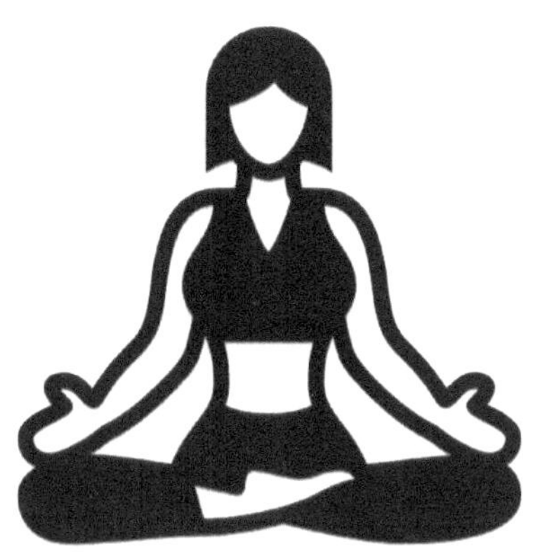

42. Regular Practice of Yoga helps you in migraines & Headaches.

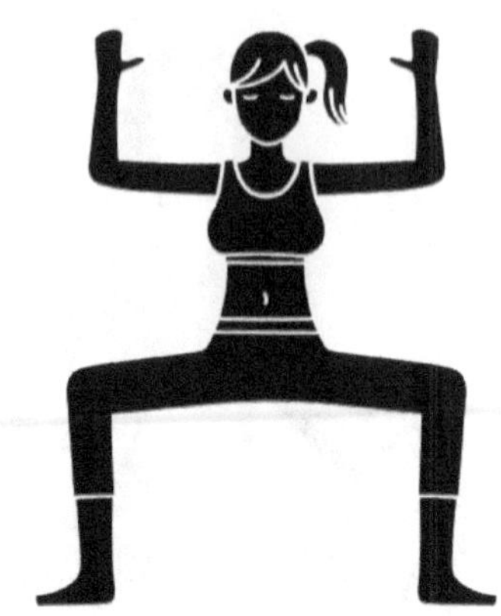

43. Certain yoga poses are believed to cleanse and balance the body's energy centers (chakras), leading to emotional and spiritual well-being.

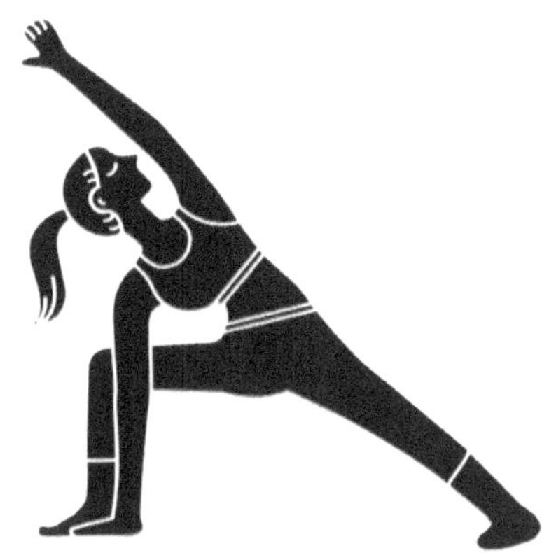

44.   Yoga strengthens bones and reduced risk of osteoporosis. Also helps in joint health and reduced risk of arthritis.

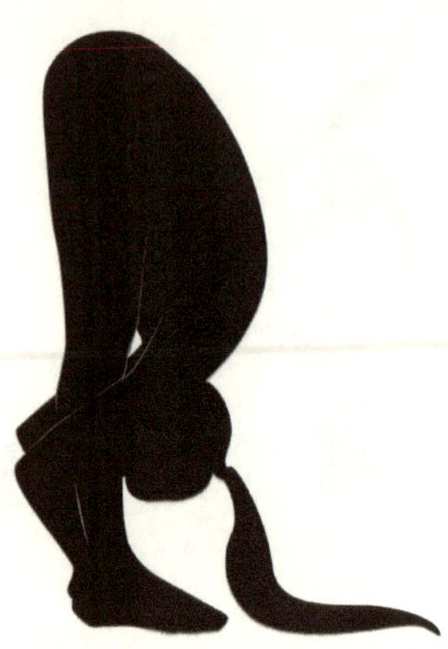

45.   It Enhances self-discipline and willpower.

46.   Some studies suggest that regular yoga practice may contribute to a longer, healthier life by reducing the risk of chronic diseases and promoting overall vitality.

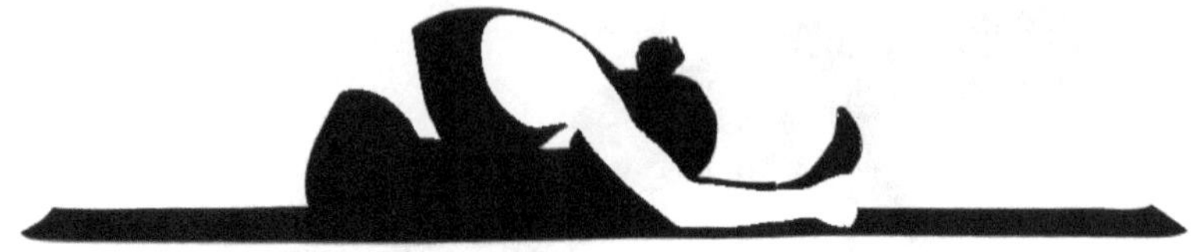

47.   Yoga Improves kidney and liver function.

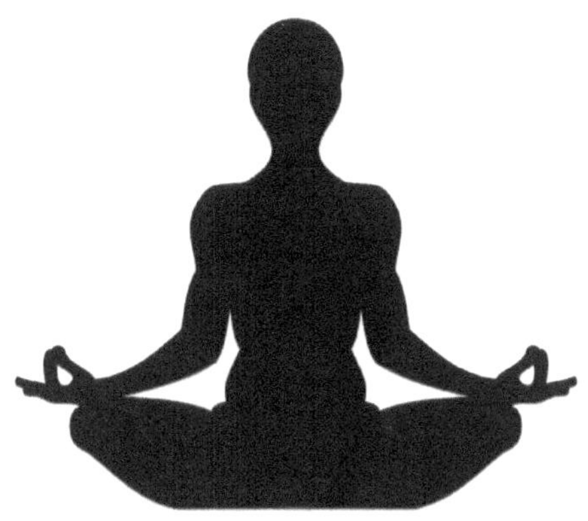

48.   Pranayam & Breathing Practices helps in increasing lung capacity and oxygenation.

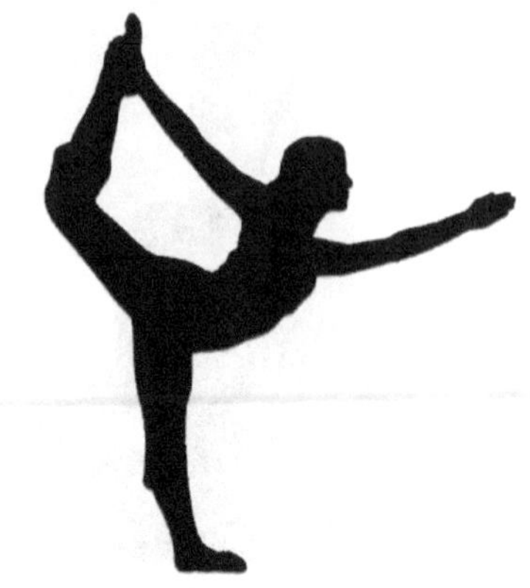

49.　Yoga is life changing, and some of us may have already experienced the shift in our thoughts and desires. What yoga also gives us is a sense of purpose – the desire to be the best version of ourselves and to make a difference in the world.

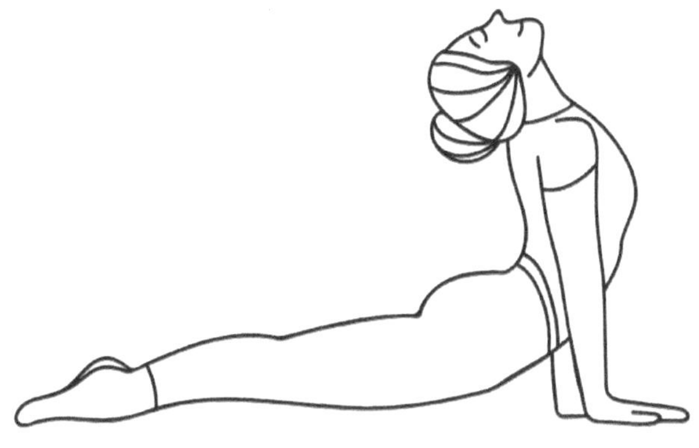

50. Practicing yoga helps the chakra energy flow with ease and allows us to clear any blockages in our body. Opening this energy flow allows you to feel subtle changes or shifts in your life.

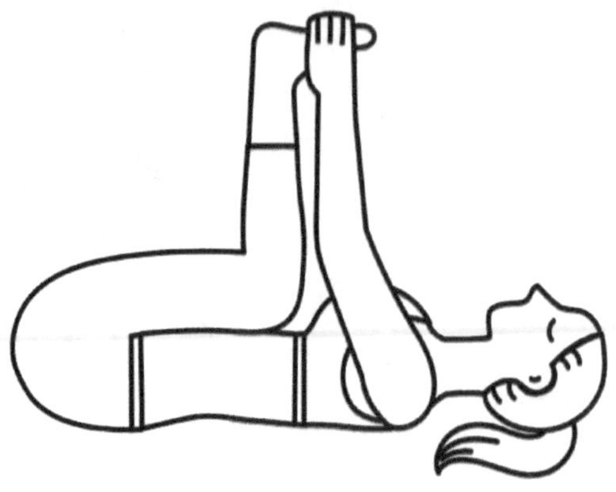

51.   Yoga Enhanced recovery from workouts and reduced muscle soreness.

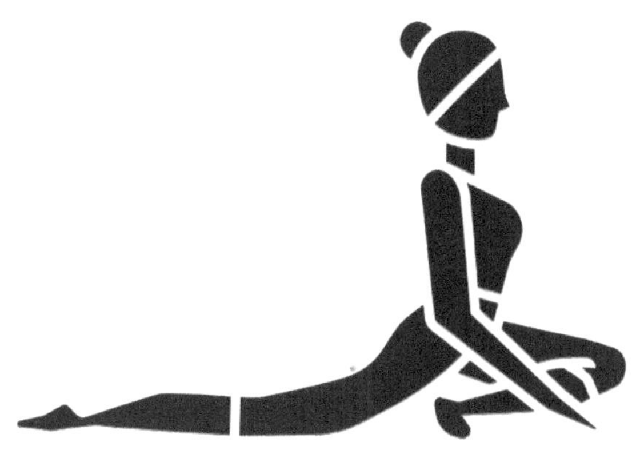

52.   Yoga helps in Reducing symptoms of menstrual cramps.

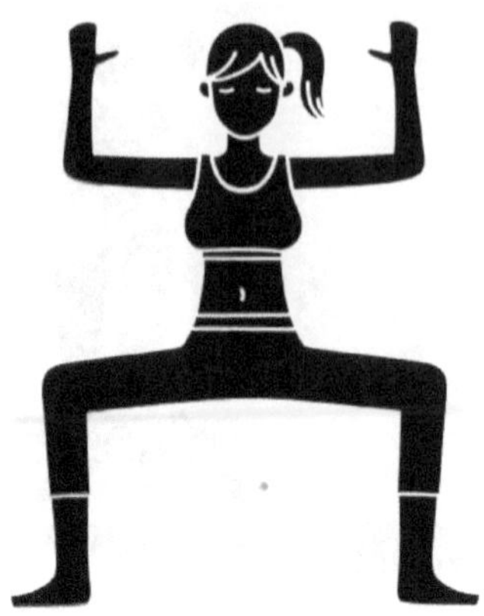

53.   Yoga Enhances fertility and reproductive health. Also Improves sexual health and libido.

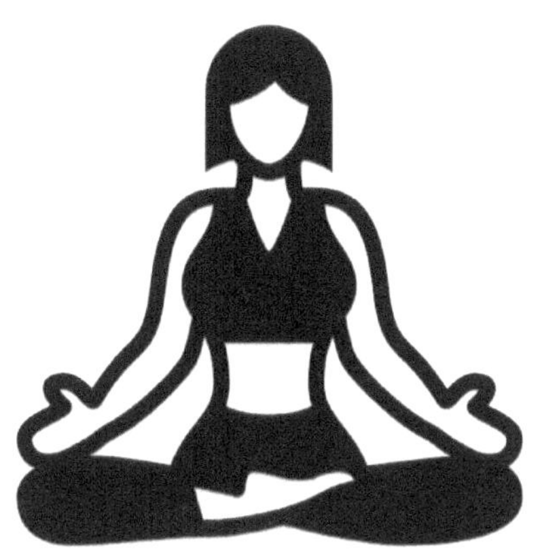

54.   Yoga provides a path for spiritual exploration and self-realization.

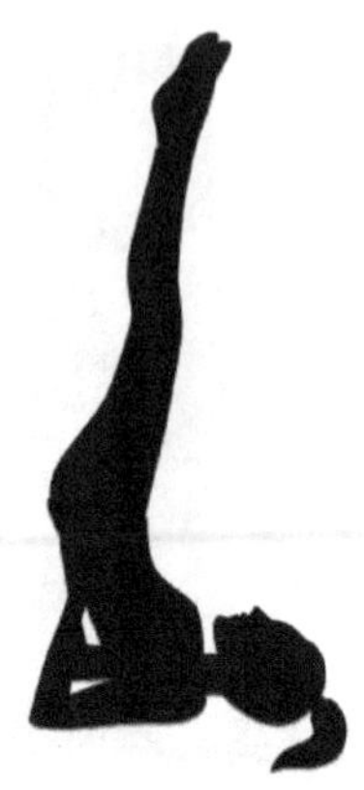

55.   Yoga can be an effective complementary approach to managing chronic pain conditions by improving flexibility and reducing muscle tension.

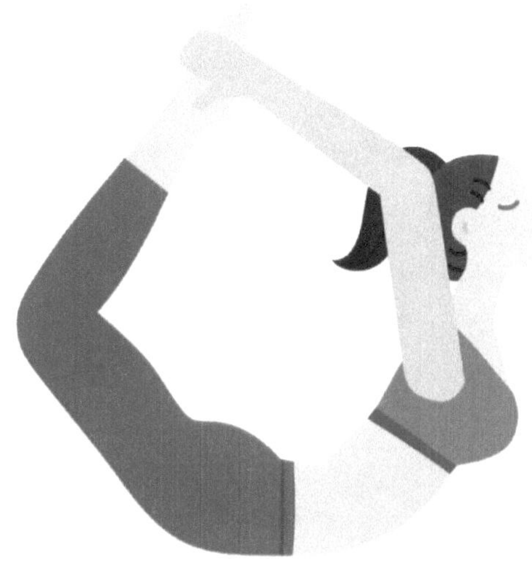

56.   It helps women in menopause by reducing pain and many other symptoms.

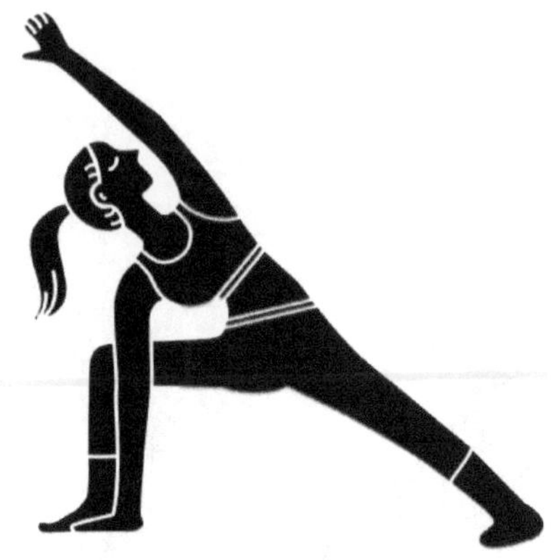

57. It Improves bladder control and reduced urinary incontinence.

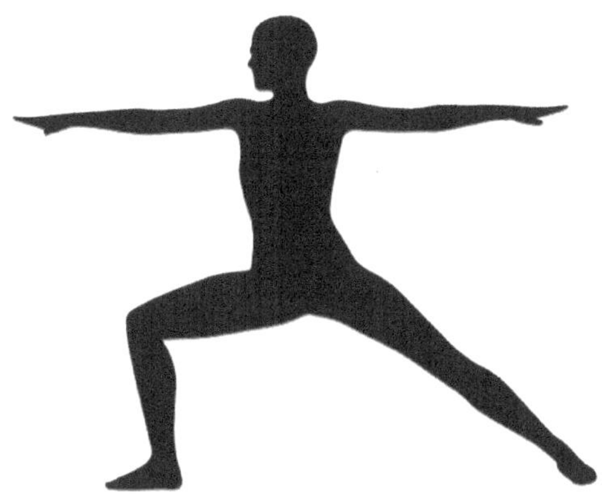

58.   Yoga reduces symptoms of allergies and respiratory conditions.

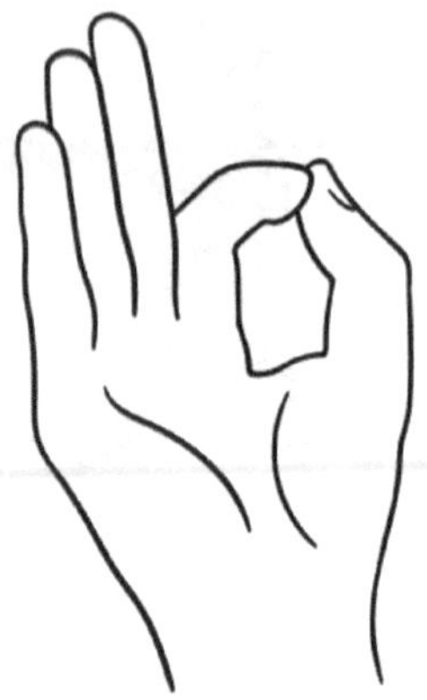

59.   Continuous practice of Face Yoga Improves eye health and reduced eye strain.

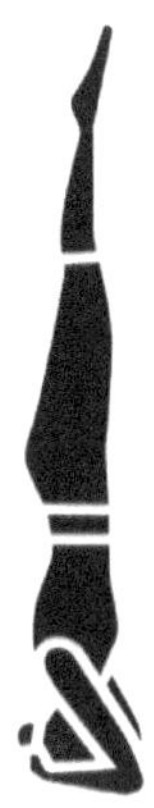

60.   Yoga Increases creativity and problem-solving skills.

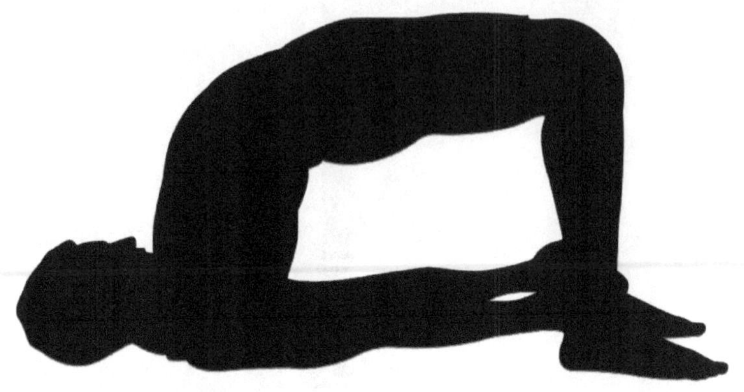

61.   Yoga improves our mental clarity and makes us more mindful.

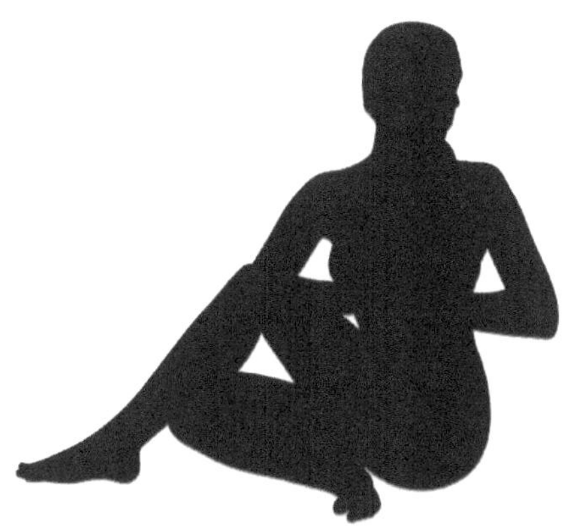

62.   Yoga Improves emotional regulation and resilience.

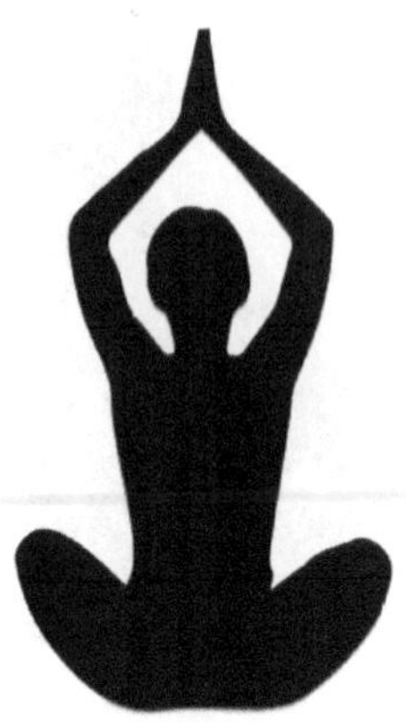

63. Yoga Reduces symptoms of PTSD and trauma-related disorders.

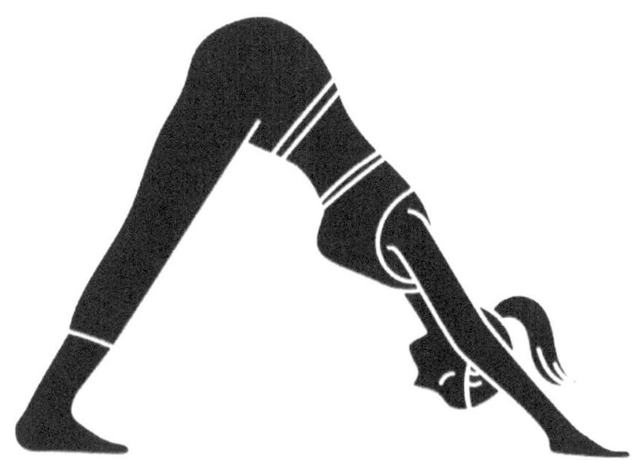

64.   Yoga improves mindful eating habits and rescues cravings for unhealthy substances.

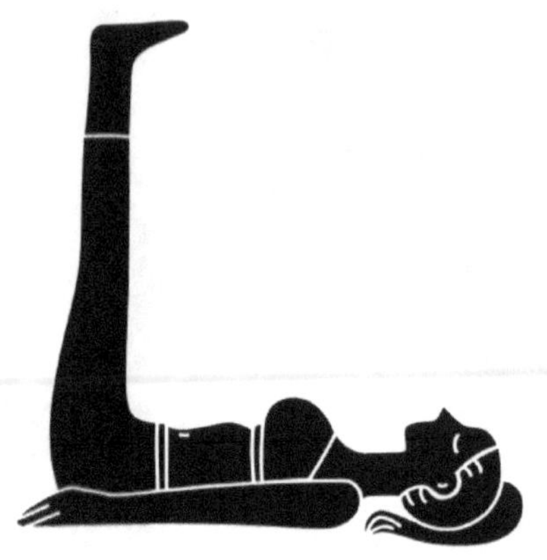

65.   Yoga helps Singers and public speakers often use yoga to improve breath control and vocal performance.

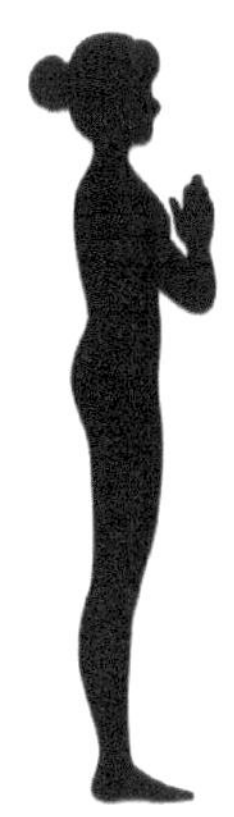

66.   Yoga reduces the risk of certain types of cancers.

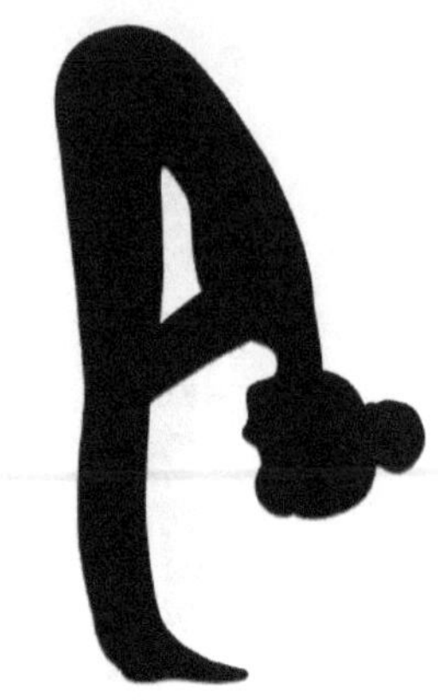

67. Yoga helps in improving liver function.

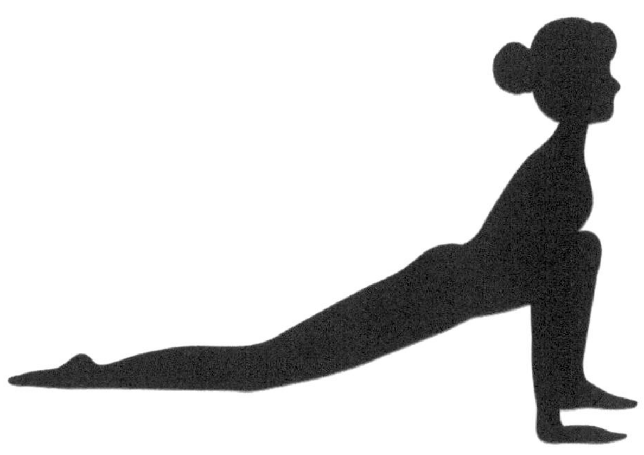

68.   Yoga encourages the practice of gratitude, fostering a more positive outlook on life.

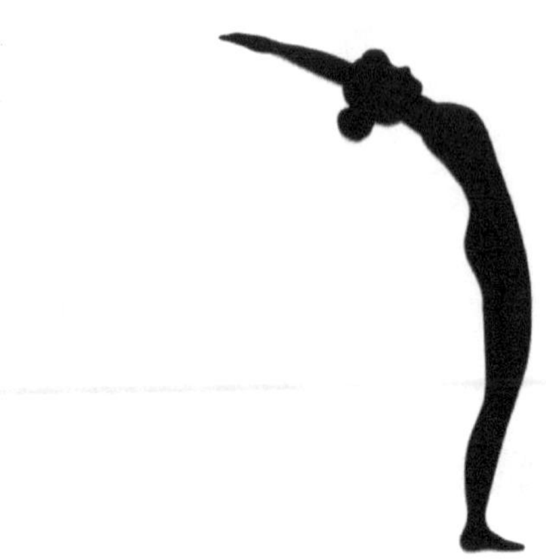

69. Yoga Reduces reliance on medications and medical interventions.

70.   Yoga improves overall quality of life.

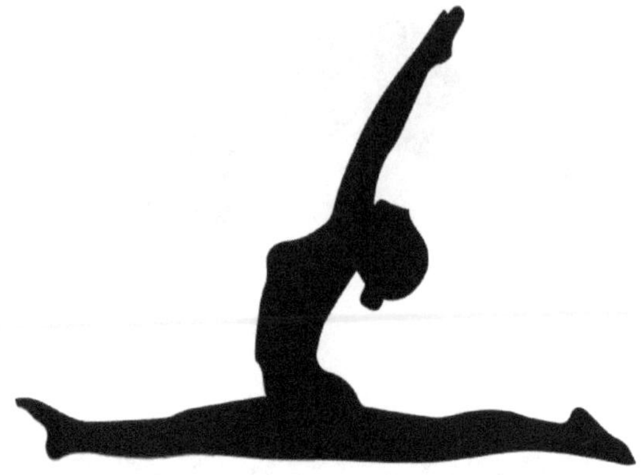

71.   Regular Practice of Yoga increases recovery from injuries or surgeries.

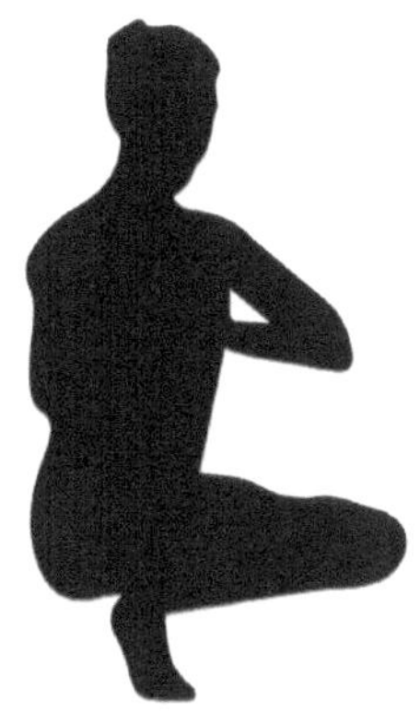

72.   Better management of fibromyalgia symptoms is possible through Yoga.

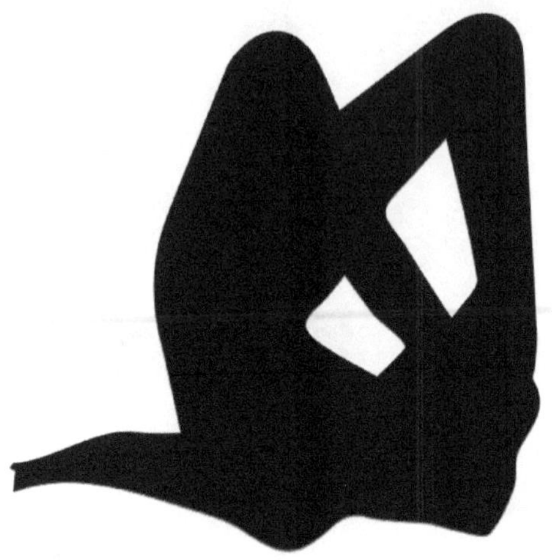

73.   Yoga reduces risks of fall by Improving balance and flexibility can reduce the risk of falls, particularly in older adults.

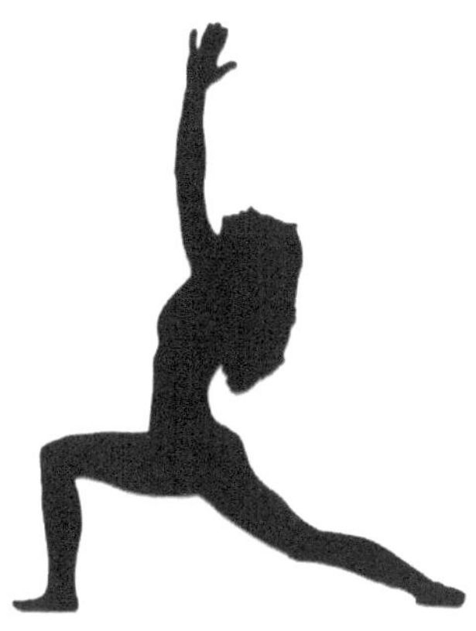

74. Yoga helps in elimination of toxins and detoxifying our body.

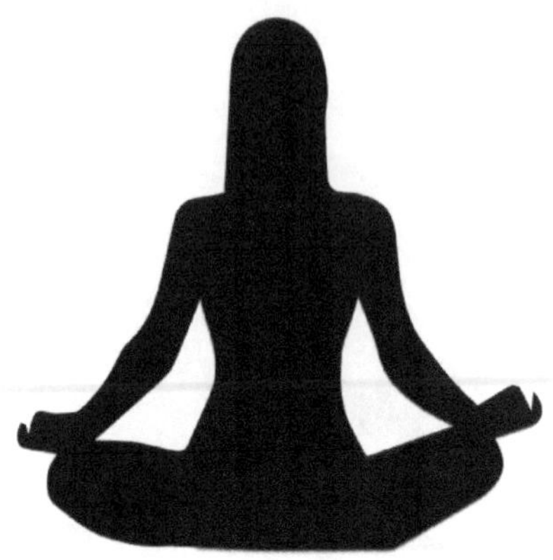

75. Yoga enhances Taste Sensation making more Mindful in eating and can heighten the enjoyment of food.

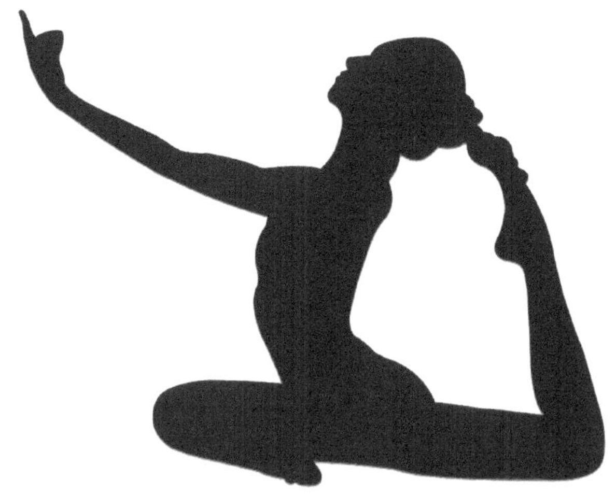

76.   Yogic practices like oil pulling can enhance oral health.

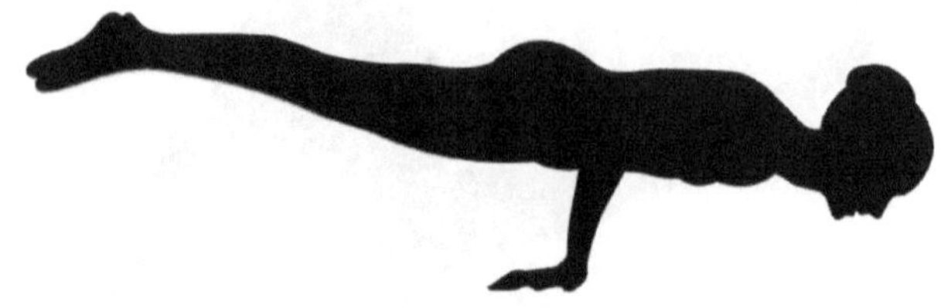

77.   Yoga makes our empathetic towards others, increases our self-compassion and self-care practices.

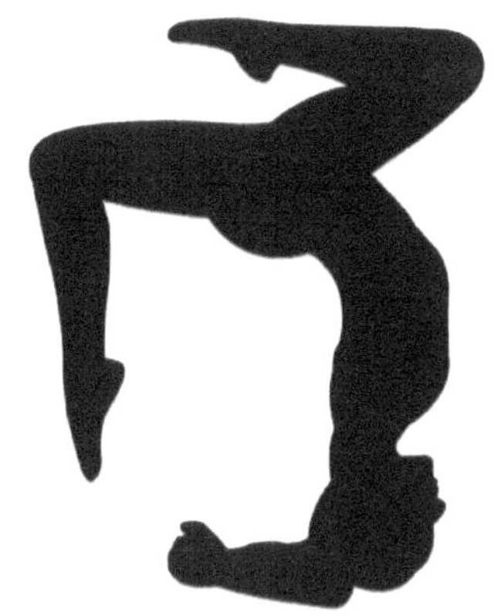

78.   Yoga can enhance your perception of depth and spatial awareness.

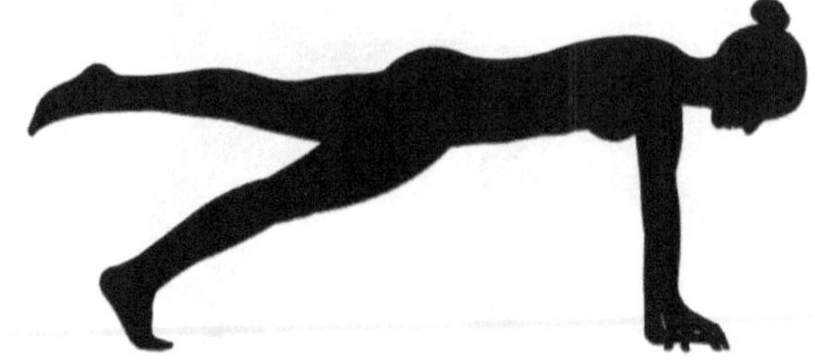

79.   Yoga increases the pain tolerance and pain management skills.

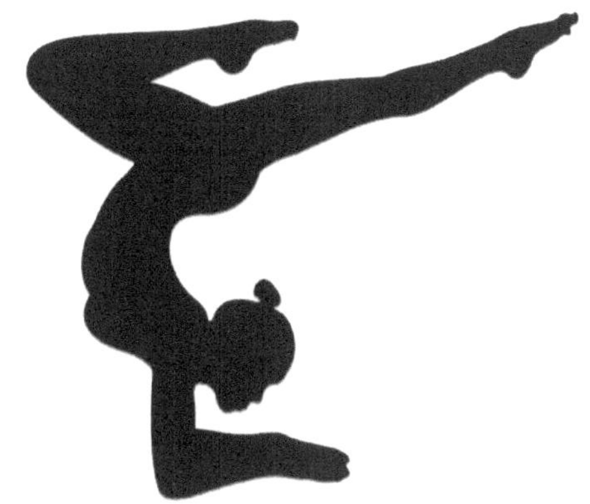

80.   Yoga practices can strengthen the muscles involved in swallowing.

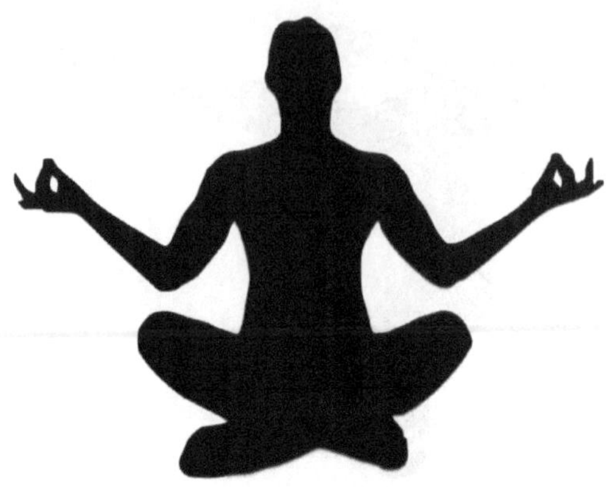

81. Yoga reduces symptoms of obsessive-compulsive disorder (OCD).

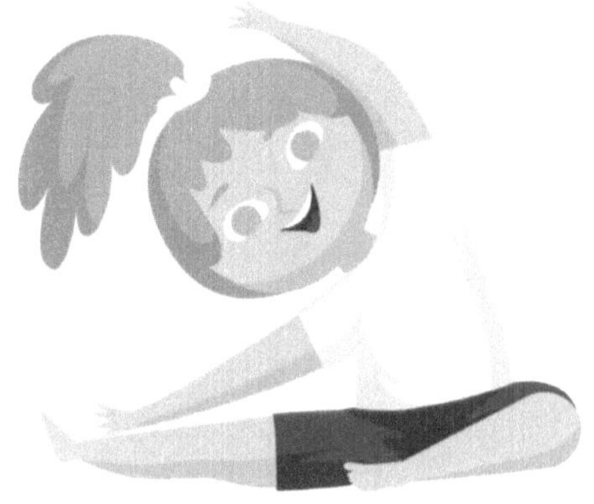

82.   Yoga helps in reducing the symptoms of attention deficit hyperactivity disorder (ADHD).

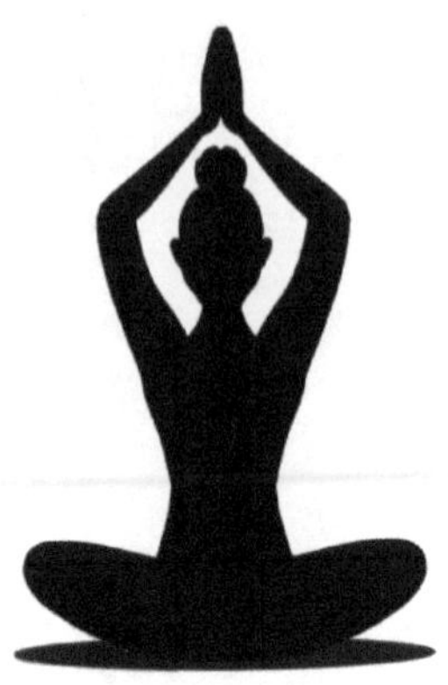

83.   Yoga improves our Intelligence Quotient & emotional intelligence.

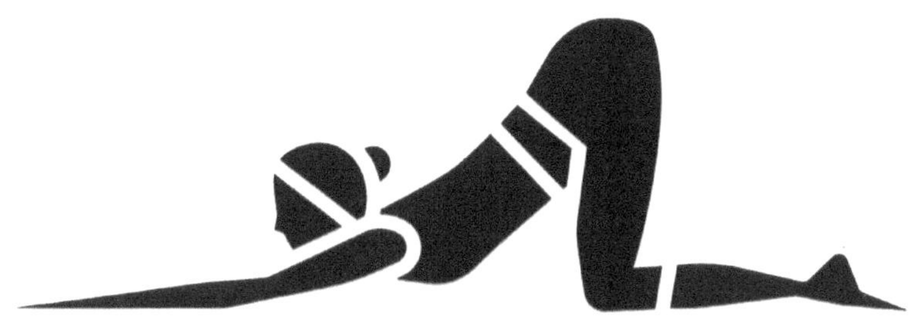

84.   Yoga and meditation can enhance the synchronization of brainwave patterns.

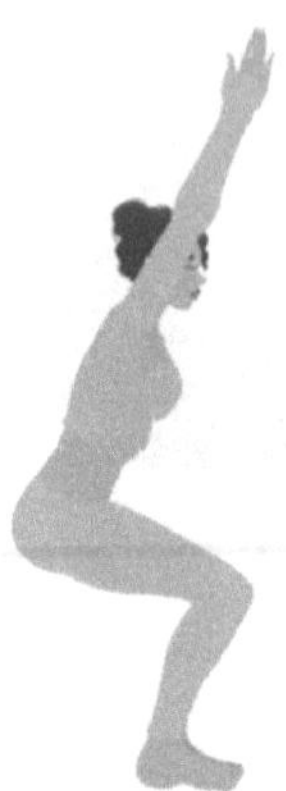

85. Better focus and awareness developed through yoga can enhance driving skills.

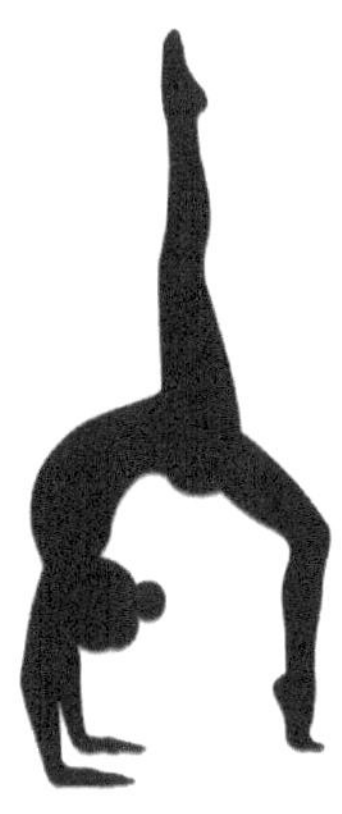

86. Yoga reduces the risk of age-related macular degeneration (AMD).

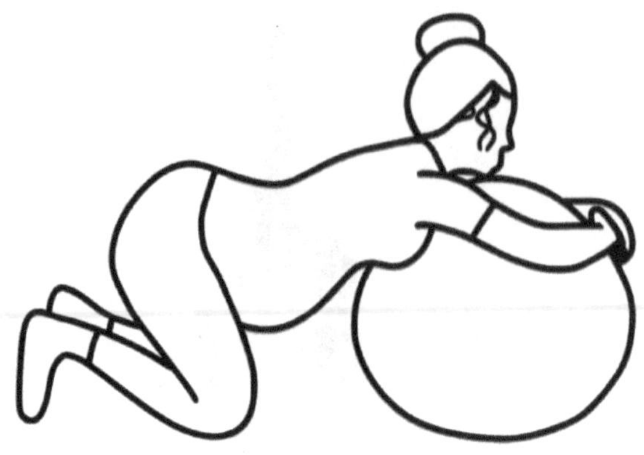

87. Prenatal yoga can increase pain tolerance during labor.

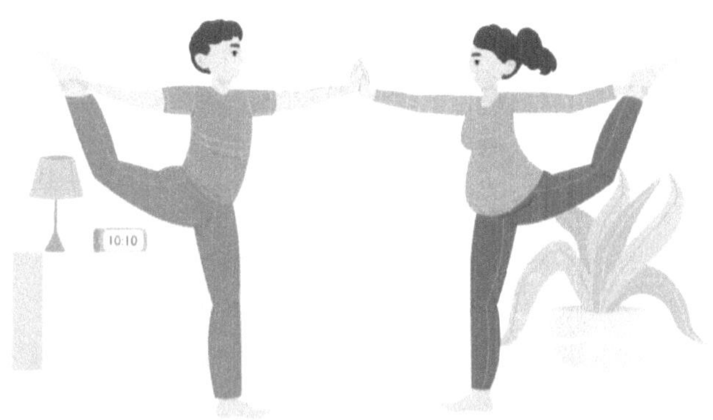

88. Yoga alleviates athletic recovery time.

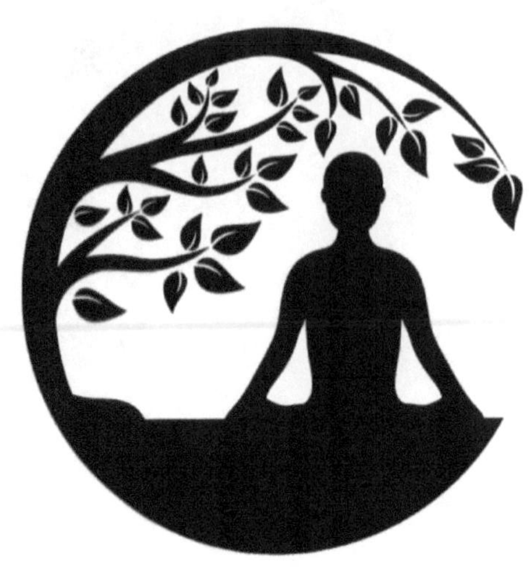

89. Yoga can improve concentration, focus and reaction times for archery, boxing, for gamers etc.

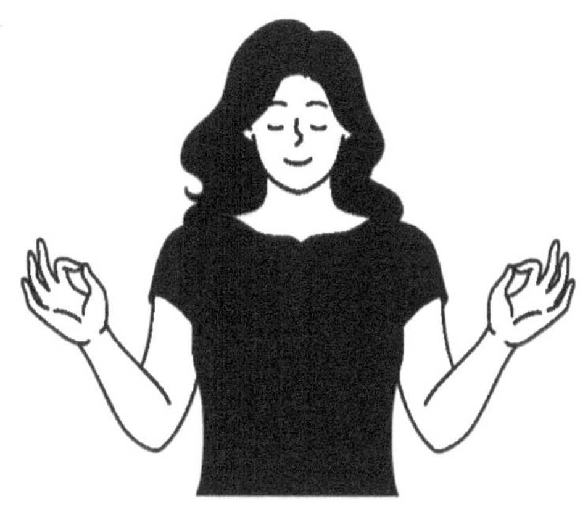

90.   YOGIC BREATHING
is less susceptibility to minor illness such as bronchitis and asthma.

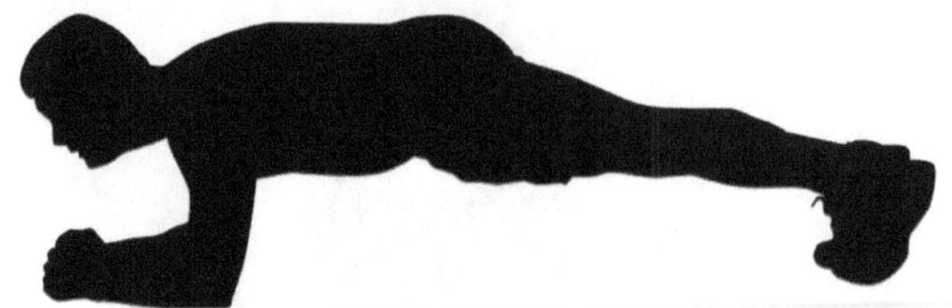

91.   Yoga can strengthen the core muscles crucial for dance.

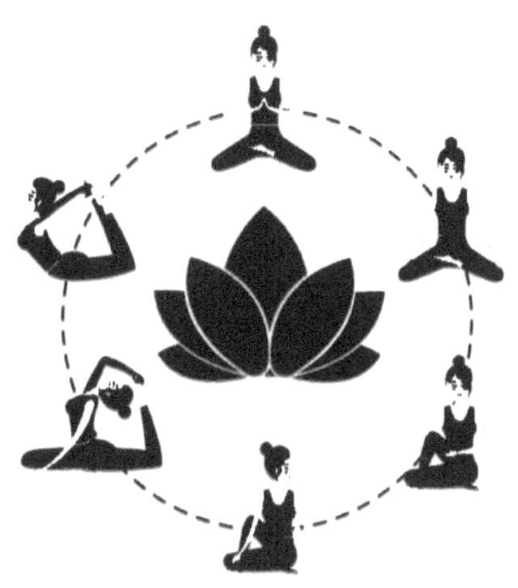

92.   Yogic Breathing
Improved vitality, less fatigue.

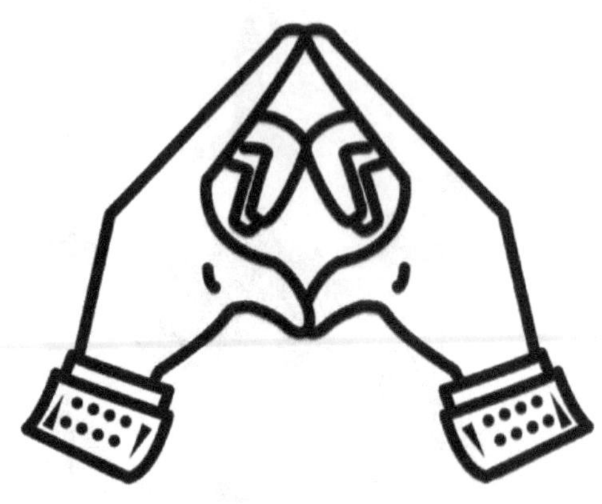

93.   By daily practising Yogic mudras it helps in regaining health and no medication in Mudras. Therefore there is no reaction of chemicals.

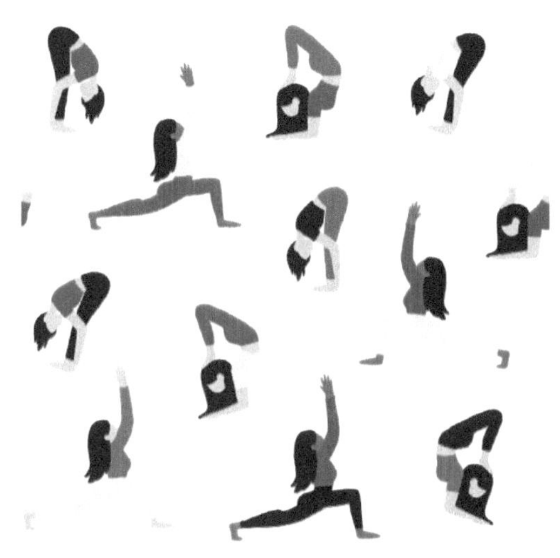

94.   Yoga can enhance flexibility and balance for martial arts, cyclists and reducing risk of injury.

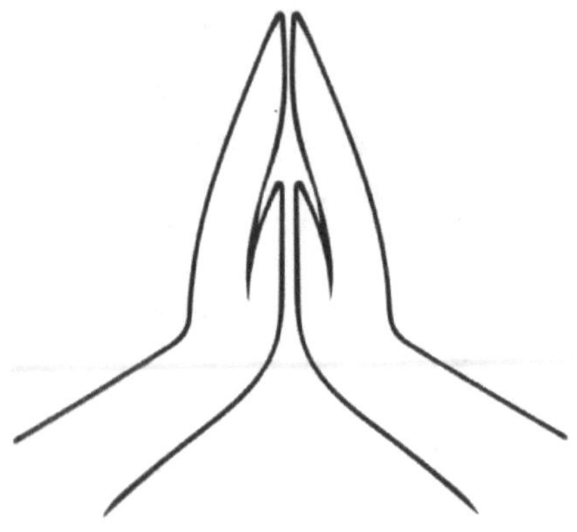

95. Yoga can improve arm and wrist strength and flexibility.

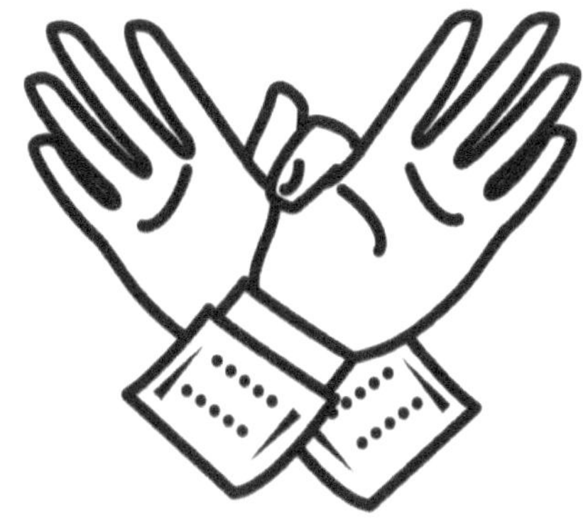

96. Better blood circulation through yoga can promote healthier hair and a natural shine.

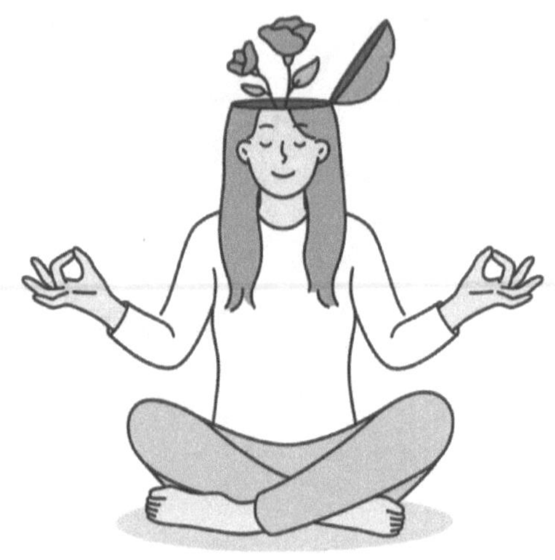

97. Yoga's focus on mindfulness can improve your ability to remember people's names.

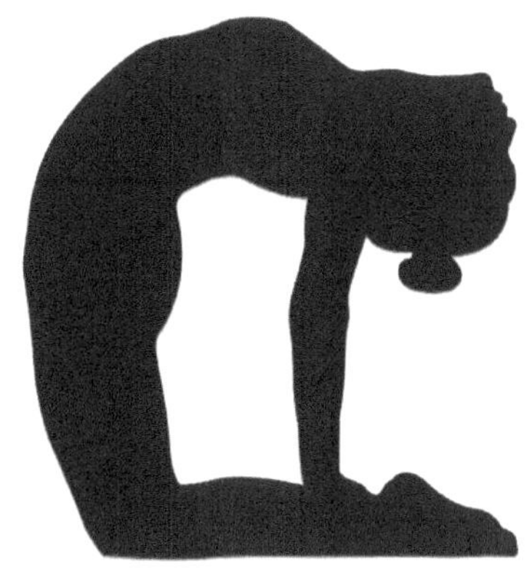

98.   Yoga can help reduce the hunched posture often associated with phone use.

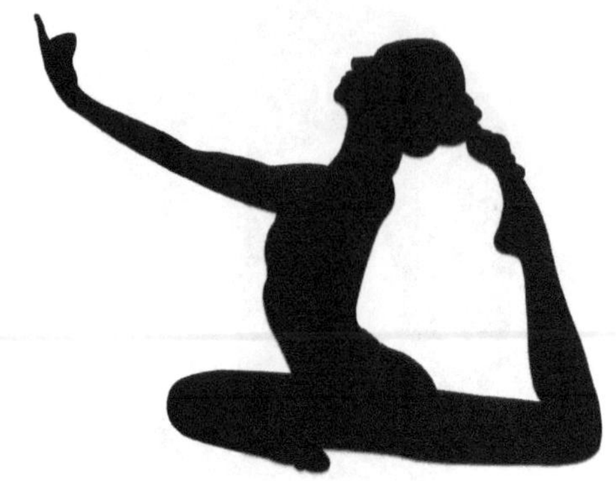

99. Yoga's focus on conquering fears can help with acrophobia (fear of heights).

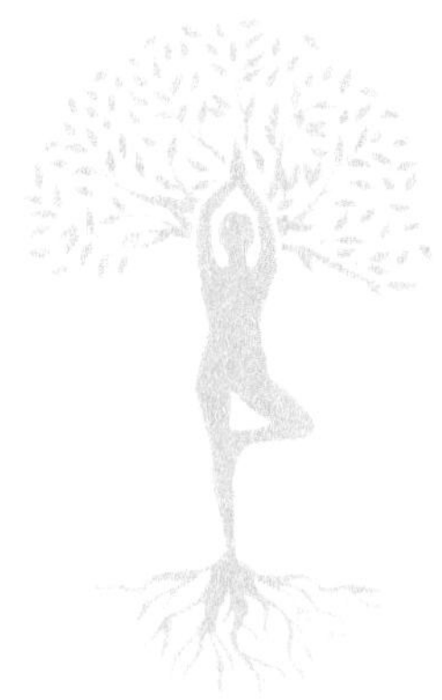

100. Yogic Mudras being universal they can be performed anywhere and any time and by anybody

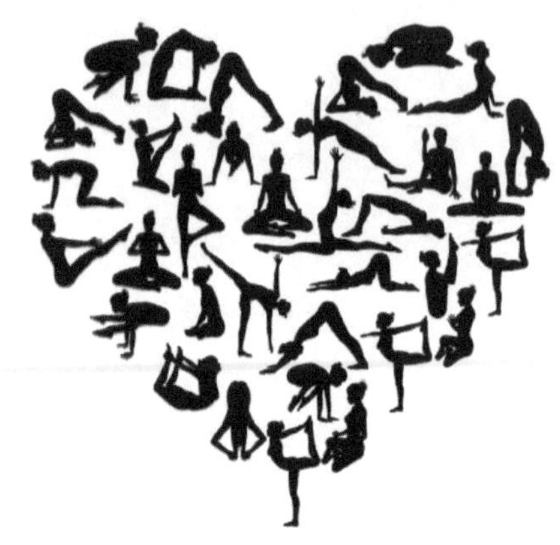

101. Continuous Practice of Yoga for years will lead us to our ultimate goal that is Divination.

Do you know any more friends in your circle you would like to share these affirmations? List their name below.

1. ....

2. ....

3. ....

4. ....

5. ....

6. ....

7. ....

8. ....

9. ....

10. ....

Varuna Sacheti embodies expertise in the realm of fitness and exercise, particularly standing out as a highly skilled practitioner of yoga. Her role as a motivational fitness enthusiast is undeniable, and her videos have consistently provided the encouragement I needed to place fitness at the forefront of my own life. Varuna's mastery of yoga is truly commendable, and her efforts to promote its significance resonate strongly. Here's to wishing her the utmost success in her endeavour to share the importance of yoga in people's lives through this book.

- ***Khushboo Bhavesh Chotaliya***
Author & Wedding Decor Exporter
@KhushbooBChotaliya

Varuna, based in Lokhandwala, Mumbai, is a highly skilled yoga instructor known for her expertise in the field. She is renowned for her enthusiastic approach to wellness and her unique teaching style. Varuna's teaching philosophy revolves around first applying her extensive knowledge and practical experience before imparting it to her students. This hands-on approach ensures that her students receive instruction that is not only informed but also deeply rooted in practical application.

- ***Yogesh M.A.***
Digital Leadership Trainer
@brandyouyear

Varuna is a yoga instructor with a difference Her dedication and patience for teaching yoga for perfect health is exemplary. She is a true fitness enthusiast in the absolute essence of it and keeps inspiring everyone with her consistent work out sessions. Believing and upholding good health through the mantra of "Yoga se hi hoga" makes her live upto her mission of fitness Keep up the good work!

- ***Chandrani Bagdey***
Author &Lifestyle Management Coach
@chandranibagdey

Meet Varuna, a beacon of fitness and discipline. With unwavering dedication, she embraces each day with a commitment to exercise, never allowing excuses to derail her routine. Her contagious enthusiasm ripples through those around her, inspiring everyone to push their limits and embrace a healthier lifestyle. In her presence, excuses crumble, replaced by a shared determination to chase wellness goals. Varuna's ability to motivate effortlessly transforms every interaction into a step towards a fitter, more disciplined life.

\- ***Sneha Kalbag***
Social Event Planner
@kalbagsneha

Varuna mam is an incredibly focused and committed individual. Her humility and kindness shine through, serving as a great example. She's a source of motivation for my fitness goals, communicating more through her actions than words. Wishing her all the best.

\- ***Vivek Trivedi***
Founder – CureForSure.com
@vivektrivediofficial

Varuna Sacheti has been an inspiration for many. When it comes to fitness and health, she is super passionate about yoga and has been training many people with her vast experience in yoga and fitness. Wishing you a prosperous future ahead.

\- ***Neha Sawant***
Author & Sales Expert
@nehasawant.ig